The cellular regeneration impact on cancer

By Dr. Lucy Coleman

For permissions or further inquiries, please contact:

support@lifebossnetwork.com |

10 9 8 7 6 5 4 3 2 1

ISBN: 978-1-949545-24-1

The cellular regeneration impact on cancer

A guide on how to use emerging techniques to fight cancer

Dr. Lucy Coleman

COLEMAN PUBLISHING

Coleman Publishing

In loving memory of Norberto Costa, Elina Aguiar and Derrick Coleman, remarkable souls whose strength, courage, and legacy continue to inspire. This book is also dedicated to every brave fighter facing the battle against cancer. You are not alone. Let's rise, resist, and reclaim life—together.

"Natural forces within us are the true healers of disease"

- Hippocrates

Contents

Introduction

For many years now, I have worked closely with patients navigating one of life's most daunting diagnoses: cancer. Each person I've supported has reinforced a truth I hold close—there is a reason for everything. My mother would say this often when I was growing up, and with time, experience, and deep introspection, I've come to believe her. But the meaning behind that phrase has evolved profoundly for me.

I trained as a medical doctor and, early on, discovered a deep passion for reproductive medicine and embryology. My fascination with the miracle of life led me to build a successful fertility practice. I devoted myself wholeheartedly to helping others bring life into the world—a dream I visualized, worked tirelessly toward, and ultimately lived out.

I believed I had found my purpose. My days were filled with meaning, and I was grateful for the work I did.

But life, in its mysterious wisdom, redirected my path.

There was a quiet voice inside me—a curious, scientific, and perhaps even spiritual whisper—nudging me to look deeper. To expand. I loved my fertility work, but something within me was urging me to explore more, to understand the body in ways my conventional training had not prepared me for. At the time, I didn't fully comprehend this call. But everything became clearer when I faced my own unexpected health crisis.

A brain issue—sudden, frightening, and unexplained—forced me to stop everything.

I walked out of the hospital with a shopping bag full of medications, each one aimed at managing a symptom. The list of side effects for each drug was longer than the benefits they promised. Something inside me rebelled. I held that bag, looked at it, and asked myself a question that would change everything:

"Is this really what healing looks like?"

At that moment, I made a bold decision. I threw away the medications and committed myself to a new path—one rooted not in suppression, but in understanding. Not in numbing the body, but in listening to it.

I stepped away from the world I knew and dove into an exploration of medicine that transcended prescriptions. I wanted to understand the true essence of healing—not just at the physical level, but at the emotional, psychological, energetic, and cellular levels.

This journey led me to a profound realization: we have been conditioned to treat symptoms as enemies, rather than messages.

Symptoms are the body's language. They are how it tells us something is off balance. They are not random; they are not nuisances. They are signals—wise, intricate, and precise. When we ignore them, or worse, suppress them without understanding their root cause, we silence an inner alarm system designed to protect us.

I had been doing it wrong. Not intentionally, but by following a system that teaches us to compartmentalize the body and treat organs, tissues, and systems in isolation. Medical school gave me a foundational understanding of anatomy and pathology, but it was incomplete. I had never been taught to see the body as a deeply interconnected web of physical, emotional, energetic, and even spiritual intelligence.

As I began to explore integrative and functional approaches to medicine, I encountered a community of professionals—physicians, scientists, healers, researchers—who were asking the same questions I was. People who believed that the human body was more than a machine and that healing required more than medication.

I learned about the connection between trauma and illness. I studied the science of epigenetics, neuroplasticity, detoxification, and energy medicine. I discovered how emotions like grief, fear, and anger can be stored at the cellular level, influencing health and disease.

And slowly, I began to piece together a different kind of healing model—one that recognized the intelligence of the body and the incredible regenerative capacity of our cells.

This awakening led me to develop Hypnocell®, a methodology that allows access to the subconscious mind and cellular programming through hypnosis. It helps identify and neutralize the root cause of disease by tapping into the body's own repair mechanisms. Using this approach, I began helping patients not only with fertility but with chronic illnesses—and eventually, with cancer.

As I deepened my research and clinical experience, I became more and more fascinated with the concept of cellular regeneration. I began to ask bold questions:

- What if our cells can be taught to return to balance?

- What if disease is not a punishment, but a miscommunication?

- What if healing is possible—not just symptom relief—but real, cellular-level healing?

The more I worked with patients and listened to their stories, the more I saw patterns. Patients who had suppressed emotions for decades. Patients who had ignored their bodies' early warnings. Patients who, once they made lifestyle changes, embraced detox practices, rewired their thought patterns, and engaged in deeper inner healing, experienced remarkable turnarounds—even in so-called "hopeless" cases.

I came to understand that cancer is not a random curse—it is, in many cases, a metabolic, emotional, and environmental disease. It does not happen overnight. It builds silently, over years, fed by inflammation, toxicity, unresolved trauma, poor nutrition, stress, and disconnection from the body.

The good news is that the body remembers how to heal. When we provide the right conditions—mentally, physically, emotionally, and spiritually—it begins to restore itself.

My mission with this book is to share what I've learned and help empower you with a new understanding of healing. This is not a book of empty promises. It is a guide grounded in science, experience, and deep compassion. Whether you are a patient, a caregiver, or someone simply looking to understand the bigger picture of health, this book will serve you.

You'll discover:

- Why understanding the root cause of cancer is essential

- How your cellular environment shapes your health

- What role nutrition, movement, detox, and emotional healing play in regeneration

- How to use mindset, meditation, and subconscious programming as powerful healing tools

- What you can do right now—regardless of your diagnosis—to begin healing from within

This is not about abandoning conventional medicine. It's about expanding your options and recognizing that you are not powerless in your health journey. Whether you are using chemotherapy, alternative therapies, or both, this book will help you build an integrative healing roadmap that honors your entire being.

I want you to know something before we begin:

You have the power to heal.

It's not magic. It's biology, consciousness, and commitment working in harmony. It's your innate intelligence, activated with intention and supported by the right tools and information.

This is the book I wish every patient could have when they hear the words "you have cancer." This is the guide I wish had existed when I faced my own health crisis. And this is the message I want the world to hear:

Healing is possible. Regeneration is real. And your body is wiser than you've ever been taught to believe.

Quick fixes do not work

One of the greatest concerns I have with conventional Western medicine is its tendency to address signs and symptoms without fully understanding their deeper, integrative meaning. In many cases, symptoms are viewed as the problem to eliminate, rather than as important messages from the body—a sophisticated internal alarm system trying to draw our attention to deeper imbalances.

Instead of silencing these signals with pharmaceuticals, we should be asking: *Why is the body sending this signal? What is it trying to tell me?* Only when we answer those questions can we begin to heal from the inside out.

Silencing symptoms backfires

The human body is not a collection of isolated parts—it is a beautifully interconnected system composed of cells that carry memory, intelligence, and the potential for regeneration. Each cell is influenced by internal and external factors: environment, nutrition, thought patterns, stress levels, emotional state, and even unhealed trauma. These factors all play a role in how our cells behave—whether they choose to repair and regenerate or degenerate and decline.

From the very beginning of our lives, our cells are imprinted with experiences. These imprints form a biological memory that shapes not only our physical health but our susceptibility to illness. I realized that our daily actions, even those we consider insignificant, accumulate over time and influence how our cells respond to the environment. Chronic illness, in this view, is not random—it is often the culmination of years of cellular confusion, toxicity, and miscommunication.

My work in human reproduction and embryology gave me a unique window into this phenomenon. I observed how early-stage embryos developed, divided, and responded to their environment. If an embryo was exposed to a stressful or toxic setting, it would often show signs of arrested development, such as poor cellular division and fragmentation. But when cultivated in a nurturing, peaceful environment—with calming music and gentle care—these embryos developed faster, healthier, and more harmoniously.

That experience reshaped my entire understanding of medicine. I saw firsthand that cells listen to their environment. Genetics are only part of the equation—epigenetics, the environment in which genes are expressed, plays a powerful role in determining outcomes. Even couples with excellent clinical prognosis sometimes produced poor-quality embryos when under high stress. Conversely, couples with seemingly low odds sometimes produced excellent embryos when supported with calm, nurturing care.

This observation inspired me to create a new methodology that would focus on supporting cells—not just in embryos, but throughout the human body. I developed a system that exposed embryos to soothing sound environments and allowed patients to speak to their embryos while they were in the incubators. The results were astonishing—embryo quality improved, fragmentation decreased, and pregnancy rates increased.

That's when it clicked: if these early cells could be influenced by their environment so profoundly, why wouldn't all cells in the body respond the same way?

So I began exploring how to "communicate" with cells at a deeper level. That's when I developed Hypnocell®, a groundbreaking technique that uses clinical hypnosis to access the subconscious mind and speak directly to the cellular memory. Through this method, I guide patients to uncover the emotional and energetic roots of their disease, reprogram harmful beliefs, and support the body's innate regenerative capacity.

The results were remarkable. Fertility outcomes improved significantly. Patients experienced better hormonal balance, less inflammation, and deeper emotional clarity. And then came my first cancer patient.

Although I had always found oncology fascinating, I had never pursued it formally. My heart belonged to embryology. But cancer came knocking on my door in the form of a brave woman who had been a fertility patient and later developed the disease. She had already endured so much—and she was exhausted by the ongoing barrage of conventional treatments. She needed a different approach.

That case changed everything. I dove into the study of oncology with renewed purpose, combining conventional knowledge with research into cellular healing, nutrition, detoxification, self-hypnosis, and emotional release. I studied survivors who had overcome stage IV cancers with natural therapies and mindset shifts. I read obsessively, traveled for training, and immersed myself in this new world of integrative healing.

And the stories I discovered inspired me deeply.

There were patients who had reversed autoimmune conditions, degenerative diseases, and yes—even terminal cancer—by shifting their diets, healing old emotional wounds, practicing daily movement, and retraining their minds. I began applying these principles with my own patients, developing a complete healing protocol that addressed body, mind, and spirit.

I founded LifeBoss Health, a comprehensive healing program designed to help individuals take back control of their physical, emotional, and spiritual health. The first steps involve deep subconscious work to identify the root cause of the disease, followed by targeted detoxification, physical activity, emotional processing, and mindfulness practices. This is not a quick-fix approach—it's a **complete lifestyle transformation.**

And it works.

One of the most impactful stories I can share is about a patient with **stage IV lung cancer**. After 22 chemotherapies and 2 immunotherapies, he was told there was nothing more to be done. He was given three months to live and sent to palliative care. He came to me as a last resort.

Eight years later, he is thriving.

He changed everything—his diet, his routines, his beliefs. He committed to the Hypnocell® process, integrated the LifeBoss protocol, and over time, began to witness profound improvements. He regained energy, clarity, and a deep joy for life. He remarried, moved to the coast, and now runs a successful e-commerce business from his seaside home.

His transformation wasn't magic. It was the result of commitment, self-responsibility, and trust in the process. He became the proof I needed. And now I see this pattern again and again in patients who are ready to heal on all levels.

This is why I am writing this book.

Because self-healing through cellular regeneration is real. Because cancer is not simply a genetic mutation or a stroke of bad luck—it is often the product of a long-neglected metabolic, emotional, and environmental imbalance. And because the body has the capacity to return to health if we give it the conditions it needs to do so.

If you or someone you love is facing cancer, I want you to know: you are not helpless. There are tools, techniques, and pathways available to support you—not just in fighting the disease, but in creating a life of vibrant, sustained health.

Houston, we have a problem—And it's time to fix it

One of the most striking things I've heard from my patients over the years—many of them facing a cancer diagnosis—is this: *"I knew something was wrong. I just didn't want to believe it."* Or *"I saw it coming. My lifestyle was out of control."*

This awareness, although delayed, is powerful. When a patient begins to take responsibility for their actions—or inactions—it places them a few steps ahead on the healing journey. It signals a shift away from denial, and toward transformation. Cancer, in most cases, does not appear without warning. It is not random chaos. There is always a cause. And in this book, I will help you uncover it.

Throughout my years of giving lectures, leading workshops, and working with cancer patients, their families, medical doctors, and integrative practitioners, I've witnessed a recurring pattern: the turning point often comes when we identify the root cause of the disease. Not just its clinical name or stage—but the underlying imbalance that allowed it to develop. When the root is uncovered, everything changes. It becomes the foundation for real healing, and the path for cellular regeneration is revealed.

The challenge? Our logical mind—what I call our "left-brain filter"—often blocks new information that doesn't align with our traditional beliefs. It's a safety mechanism, but also a limitation. However, once we experience results that defy what we've been told is possible, the mind opens, the walls come down, and the healing begins.

That's why I invite you to stay open. Commit to trying these tools and steps with consistency. Don't rush. Just follow the process. The body will respond—it always does. Healing is not magic; it's biology. Cause and effect.

And here's one of the most empowering truths you'll find in this book: you hold the power to heal yourself.

No one will heal you *for* you. I'm not here to take control of your treatment. What I will do is guide you. I will show you how to reconnect with the wisdom of your own body, your own cells, your own mind. That's where the transformation begins. And that's where your power lives.

You'll discover how cellular regeneration offers the body a second chance to return to balance. But let me be clear: just as cancer takes time to develop, healing also takes time. This isn't a quick fix or a magic pill. It's a deeply layered process that, when done right, leads to long-lasting results.

If you're looking for real change, if you're committed to taking your power back and walking the path of self-healing, then this book was written for you. If you're simply searching for a fast solution, a pharmaceutical promise, or a bandage approach, then you may need to come back to this book later—when you're truly ready.

I will walk you through everything. Step by step. Gently and clearly. Your only task is to stay open, stay consistent, and allow your mind and body to trust the process.

Let's face it—just hearing the word "cancer" sparks fear in almost everyone. That fear is valid, but fear without knowledge is paralyzing. The antidote is education.

Cancer is more common than ever. Every day, thousands of people receive a diagnosis, and millions more live under its shadow—physically, emotionally, mentally. It affects not only the patient, but families, communities, and even entire health systems.

This book was also created for those who are supporting someone with cancer. You may be a caregiver, a spouse, a friend, or a medical practitioner looking for answers beyond the conventional route. Here, you'll find a roadmap.

Did you know that one in four people in the United States will be diagnosed with cancer this year? That number is staggering. And a large percentage of those cases are directly related to lifestyle, nutrition, and environmental stressors.

We are what we eat, breathe, think, and feel. Chronic diseases—including cancer—are not sudden events. They are the result of long-term nutritional deficiencies, emotional stress, toxic exposure, and the suppression of symptoms instead of addressing root causes.

Nutritional therapy, for instance, is one of the most powerful tools we have. Yet it's often dismissed in mainstream cancer treatment. Meanwhile, treatments like chemotherapy and radiation—ironically—are listed as carcinogenic themselves by the International Agency for Research on Cancer.

Drugs like Tamoxifen, commonly used to treat breast cancer, are classified in Group 1 carcinogens. And while these treatments may temporarily reduce tumor size or extend life expectancy, they often do so at the cost of long-term cellular damage: DNA disruption, inflammation, oxidative stress, immune suppression, and microbiome destruction—all known to support cancer growth.

That's why integrative oncology is gaining ground. These practitioners are pioneering a balanced approach—combining the best of conventional medicine with nutritional therapy, detox protocols, movement, mindfulness, and cellular regeneration techniques like the ones I share in this book.

So, should you choose the clinical path or the natural path? That decision is yours. I'm simply here to offer knowledge, options, and a new lens. My goal is to empower you with evidence, logic, science, and results-based techniques that can work alongside or independent from conventional treatments.

Many people avoid learning about cancer until it's too late. They wait until a diagnosis forces them to scramble for answers. But my message to you is this: *don't wait*.

Knowledge is your greatest defense. It is also your greatest tool for healing. Chronic illness is not a matter of fate. It's a message—a call to awaken.

And when that call comes, you want to be ready.

I'll also show you powerful ways to prepare your mind for healing. Optimism, visualization, and belief play a role just as vital as food and medicine. You'll learn how to train your mind to support—not sabotage—your recovery.

Whether you are newly diagnosed, supporting a loved one, or just seeking to understand more about how cancer works and how to support the body naturally, this book will serve as a guide.

Let's begin with the first chapter, where we lay the foundation of what cancer really is. You'll soon see: this isn't just about surviving—it's about reclaiming your health and thriving.

Chapter 1

Cancer is everyone's business

Cancer is a word that sparks fear, confusion, and often, a sense of helplessness. But understanding cancer begins with recognizing one crucial fact: cancer is not some mysterious force that strikes at random. It is a process—a result of deep biological shifts within the body that often reflect long-standing imbalances in our environment, lifestyle, and internal health. In other words, cancer is anyone's business. It concerns all of us.

At its core, cancer is a disease of cellular dysfunction. It arises when normal cells begin to grow and divide uncontrollably, ignoring the body's built-in mechanisms for regulation and repair. Unlike healthy cells, which follow a life cycle—growing, serving a function, and then dying in a process known as apoptosis—cancer cells bypass this system. They resist death, continue to divide, and monopolize the body's resources like oxygen and nutrients, often to the detriment of other vital tissues.

A breakdown in cellular communication

In a healthy body, cells are in constant communication, coordinating growth and repair with astonishing precision. Cancer disrupts this harmony. The result? Cells that forget how to die, lose their purpose, and begin multiplying without restraint. Over time, these rogue cells form tumors or infiltrate the bloodstream and lymphatic system, spreading throughout the body—a process known as metastasis.

The 10 hallmarks of cancer

Researchers have identified ten critical characteristics that define how cancer operates in the body. These "hallmarks" help us understand its complex behavior:

1. Sustained proliferative signalingCancer cells continuously send signals to themselves to grow, even when no growth is needed.

2. Insensitivity to anti-growth signalsThey ignore the body's natural signals that usually suppress unnecessary cell division.

3. Evasion of apoptosisCancer cells refuse to undergo programmed cell death, which is how the body normally removes malfunctioning cells.

4. Limitless replicationUnlike normal cells, which can only divide a certain number of times, cancer cells can divide indefinitely.

5. Sustained angiogenesisThey hijack the body's ability to grow new blood vessels, ensuring a constant supply of nutrients and oxygen.

6. Invasion and metastasisCancer cells can move beyond their original site, invading nearby tissues and distant organs.

7. Reprogramming energy metabolismKnown as the Warburg effect, cancer cells switch to a sugar-fermenting metabolism, even in oxygen-rich conditions.

8. Avoiding immune destructionThey develop ways to hide from or suppress the body's immune system.

9. Tumor-promoting inflammationChronic inflammation, often caused by lifestyle factors, helps fuel tumor growth.

10. Genomic instability and mutationCancer cells often have defective DNA repair mechanisms, which leads to more mutations and resistance

to treatment.

What this means

Understanding these hallmarks helps us see cancer not as a sudden event but as a gradual breakdown of systems—a biological rebellion, often decades in the making.

As an embryologist, I've spent thousands of hours observing human embryos under the microscope. I've seen firsthand how environmental conditions—warmth, vibration, light, and even music—can influence cellular behavior. Embryos exposed to calm, nurturing conditions divide beautifully. Those in stressed environments often falter, displaying fragmentation or abnormal development.

This led me to a profound realization: just like embryos, our adult cells are deeply influenced by their environment. They respond to cues—both internal and external. Cancer, then, is not simply genetic fate. It is largely environmental and metabolic. In fact, only about 5–10% of cancers are directly linked to inherited genetic mutations. The remaining 90–95%? They are shaped by diet, lifestyle, chronic stress, toxin exposure, and cellular metabolism.

Cancer is a metabolic disease

This emerging view—cancer as a metabolic disease—represents a major shift from the traditional model. It suggests that instead of just focusing on killing cancer cells (often with toxic interventions like chemotherapy), we must look at what caused those cells to go rogue in the first place.

Poor diet, lack of physical activity, chronic inflammation, gut dysbiosis, toxic chemical exposure, poor sleep, and unresolved emotional trauma—these are just some of the factors that create the perfect storm for cancer to develop.

Our modern environment is filled with carcinogenic triggers:

- Ultra-processed foods

- Artificial sweeteners and preservatives

- Pesticide-laced produce

- Endocrine-disrupting chemicals in plastics, cosmetics, and cleaning supplies

- Sedentary lifestyles

- Poor sleep hygiene

- Chronic stress and negative thinking

You don't have to look far. Even our baby powders, shampoos, and air fresheners often contain toxic ingredients. Over time, the body's systems—especially the immune system, mitochondria, and detox pathways—become overwhelmed. And once cellular damage accumulates, cancer takes root.

A personal note

When I work with embryos, I am reminded of the beauty and fragility of life at its earliest stage. The way an embryo develops is a reflection of its environment. The same is true for cancer cells—but in reverse. Cancer is what happens when our internal environment becomes toxic, imbalanced, and hostile to health.

Through my own journey—from fertility specialist to brain patient to integrative medicine practitioner—I've learned that cancer is not a death sentence. It is a wake-up call. It's the body's loudest alarm that something has gone terribly wrong, but it is also an invitation: to pause, to reflect, to heal.

A call to awareness

If we know that 90% of cancer causes are modifiable, that means we have tremendous power. We can choose what we eat, how we move, what thoughts we entertain, what chemicals we allow into our homes, and how we respond to stress.

The goal of this book is not to replace conventional care, but to offer something equally vital: awareness, hope, and tools. Tools that help you prevent cancer, reverse its progression, and support your healing journey from the inside out—through cellular regeneration, metabolic healing, and the intelligence of nature.

You don't need to wait for a diagnosis to take control of your health. Start now. Start small. Start today.

The power of willingness and the role of epigenetics in healing

When I welcomed my first cancer patient into the Cellular Regeneration Program, I already held a deep conviction that healing cancer required more than attacking cells with aggressive treatments. I believed it needed a systematic, integrative approach—one that addressed the disrupted metabolism, emotional state, and subconscious patterns that often lie at the root of disease.

This patient's willingness to undergo the program with an open heart and mind—to confront not only the physical aspects of her condition but also the subconscious wounds—was a decisive factor in her progress. Healing begins with willingness, and her courage set the tone for the profound transformation that followed.

Over the years, I've met two types of patients:

1. Those who say they want to heal, but whose actions and lifestyle choices consistently contradict that desire.

2. And those who are ready to do whatever it takes—who embrace responsibility, commit to change, and trust in the wisdom of their own body.

It's always the second group that experiences the most remarkable outcomes.

Epigenetics: your environment writes on your genes

For anyone still convinced that cancer is primarily genetic, let me introduce a transformative field: epigenetics. Epigenetics proves that genes are not destiny. Instead, our environment—what we eat, how we sleep, the thoughts we think, the emotions we suppress, the chemicals we're exposed to—can literally turn genes on or off.

In other words, our genes are the canvas, but our daily choices are the brushstrokes. Chronic disease is not just a genetic failure—it's often the result of chronic exposure to environments that do not support cellular balance.

This is the foundation of the LifeBoss Health, the system I developed to empower individuals to take back full control of their health. LifeBoss addresses the four pillars of health:

- Physical

- Mental

- Emotional

- Spiritual

When these elements are aligned, fear, doubt, and helplessness begin to dissolve. What replaces them is confidence, clarity, and inner strength. Healing becomes a choice—not something that happens to you, but something you activate.

Learning from the patients who defied the odds

Many of the first cancer patients who came to me were in terminal stages. Conventional medicine had exhausted its options and sent them home with little hope. Yet, these patients became my greatest teachers. I studied their resilience and the stubborn survival tactics of their cancer cells.

What I discovered is that cancer cells are clever, adaptable, and persistent. But they are not invincible.

Once I understood their behavior, I realized that healing came down to changing the environment that allowed those cells to thrive in the first place. If you know the enemy, you can design a strategy. If you understand the terrain, you can win the battle.

This knowledge may feel overwhelming or even shocking at first. But if you are reading this book, chances are you're already seeking a different path—a path of ownership, understanding, and empowerment.

Cancer is not just a crisis. It is an invitation to wake up. It is the body's most powerful signal that something needs to change—physically, emotionally, or spiritually. The question is: how will you respond?

You can choose denial. You can give away your power to others. Or you can rise.You can choose to stop, listen to your body, and ask:

"What are you trying to tell me?"

Your body is talking. Are you listening?

Too often, people reach a crisis point because they've spent years ignoring the whispers of their body—fatigue, inflammation, digestive issues, mood swings, chronic pain. These are not random events. They are messages. When we ignore them long enough, the body raises its voice. Sometimes, that voice is cancer.

But here's the truth: the body wants to heal. It is not working against you. It is begging you to course-correct, to realign with health. And that journey begins with accountability.

Your healing is in your hands

I teach my patients to study their disease—to become researchers of their own body. We analyze symptoms, triggers, emotional patterns, lifestyle habits, and subconscious programming. Through tools like hypnosis, meditation, and cellular dialogue, we uncover the root causes buried deep in the mind and tissues.

When we identify the emotional wounds or energetic imbalances that contributed to the illness, we then build a personalized strategy—one that uses the body's weaknesses as clues and its strengths as anchors for healing.

This approach has empowered countless patients to take the reins of their treatment, no longer relying solely on external interventions. They learned to see disease not as a punishment, but as a consequence—and more importantly, as an opportunity to transform.

A new perspective on cancer

This book is not about blame. It's about ownership.It's about showing you that even when a diagnosis seems final, you still have power. You can still influence your outcome. You can change your internal and external terrain to stop feeding the disease and start nourishing your recovery.

Yes, cancer rates are increasing. But so are stress levels, toxic exposure, emotional repression, and disconnection from nature and self. In a world that moves too fast, it's easy to lose your balance. Healing, then, is about slowing down—about reconnecting with your own wisdom and rhythm.

If you've been looking for a place to start, let this be your invitation:

- Study your terrain.

- Assess your habits.

- Create an action plan.

- Make the necessary changes.

- Reclaim your power.

Because true healing isn't just about eliminating disease—it's about becoming the conscious creator of your health and your life.

If you have a body, you can make the changes: the real impact of a cancer diagnosis

Facing a cancer diagnosis is a profound shock. Nearly everyone hears the word "cancer" and immediately thinks of mortality, uncertainty, and the stark statistics—all too often focusing on those who lose the battle rather than those who survive and thrive. Yet the emotional response to diagnosis can shape healing far more than the disease itself.

The emotional toll & how to respond

Upon diagnosis, many people experience fear, anxiety, sadness, and a sense of loss—from their former health and identity. This emotional burden also impacts relationships, finances, and daily routines.

Common symptoms include insomnia, loss of appetite, guilt, anger, and physical fatigue. Recognizing these early—rather than suppressing them—can improve both mental resilience and quality of life.

But there's hope. Individuals who adopt a proactive mindset—seeing cancer as a challenge to face and not just a threat—experience significant mental and emotional benefits. Many report what psychologists call post-traumatic growth: a renewed appreciation of life, strengthened relationships, personal growth, and new meaning—even amid hardship.

Why mindset matters

Choosing to reclaim your healing power instead of surrendering it to someone else—no matter how well-intentioned—can make a tremendous difference. Supportive relationships matter: research shows emotional and social support is vital for coping and resilience. Online communities, counseling, and organized support groups all help reduce isolation and empower patients.

When you trust in your body's potential to heal—your mind, immune system, and metabolic health—you lay the foundation for empowerment and greater engagement in your recovery. Those who approach recovery with acceptance and mental clarity tend to progress with less distress and more agency.

Your power, your choice

During early consultations, some patients ask: "Should I do chemotherapy or radiation?" My role is not to dictate—but to educate. I present the pros and cons to help you make informed decisions—and I design my integrative approach to complement your choices, whether you pursue conventional treatments or not. Evidence supports that combining mind-body practices with standard care can enhance quality of life and even improve treatment tolerance.

But recovery begins inside. A patient's belief in their own ability to heal powerfully influences outcomes. That inner conviction often correlates with more rapid progress—and greater resilience when challenges arise.

Moving forward with intention

Cancer doesn't just disrupt your body—it also interrupts your whole life. But it can also become a catalyst for transformation. Instead of devolving into fear, depression, or isolation, you can reframe the experience as an opportunity for growth, healing, and rediscovery.

If you know someone who's fighting cancer, your role is vital: offering emotional stability, consistent presence, practical help, and loving support helps reduce their burden and improve outcomes. Simple acts like listening without judgment or offering concrete help (meals, errands, transportation) can make a lasting difference.

Holistic effects of a cancer diagnosis

- Physical: fatigue, weight changes, pain, inflammation, changes to appearance such as hair loss

- Emotional: anxiety, sadness, helplessness, grief

- Psychological: identity shifts, fear of recurrence, loss of autonomy

- Social & Financial: disruptions in work, relationships, and livelihood

Yet the majority of patients I've worked with learn to navigate these challenges by using the diagnosis as a stepping stone—rather than a setback.

You are not alone

Your journey doesn't have to follow fear and discouragement. Lean into learning, self-care practices, biofeedback, nutrition, mindfulness, movement, community, and supportive therapies. Proactive coping strategies—such as acceptance, social connection, goal setting, and mindful self-compassion—can significantly improve your mental and emotional resilience.

Above all: knowledge is power. Understanding cancer—its nature, its root causes, the mental-emotional terrain it carves—helps you make deliberate, life-affirming decisions. Whether you are facing the diagnosis yourself or walking beside someone who is, learning the right information now empowers you to act, heal, and live. The chapters ahead are designed to give you that clarity and direction.

Hearing the words *"You have cancer"* is life-altering. It strikes with the weight of fear, uncertainty, and the sensation of losing control. And yet, it's a phrase being heard more and more around the world. One in two people will be diagnosed with cancer in their lifetime according to the American Cancer Society. It's no longer a rare occurrence—it's become a societal norm. But here's something we forget to talk about: many people heal from cancer. They don't just survive, they thrive. And they do it by becoming active participants in their healing.

The body doesn't lie. Before disease manifests, it whispers, then speaks, and when ignored, it screams. Cancer doesn't just arrive—it builds. It takes time. It may enter quietly, but it's always a message from the body: *"Pay attention. I need your help."*

From overwhelm to ownership

At LifeBoss Health, the first step in the healing journey is not chemotherapy or a new drug. It's working on what many overlook—the emotional and mental terrain. Your thoughts, stress levels, beliefs, fears, relationships, and inner dialogue all influence how your cells behave. Your emotional chemistry literally alters your biological responses. This is not "mind over matter"—this is *mind as matter*.

When I began this work, cancer patients would find me—not because I was an oncologist, but because they were looking for something more holistic, something that acknowledged the intelligence of their body. Over time, the number of patients increased dramatically. They came seeking a different approach, one that helped them understand how to reclaim control over their health.

Many of my patients had undergone years of stress, poor sleep, processed foods, toxic relationships, overuse of pharmaceuticals, and emotional suppression.

Cancer was the body's breaking point. But what amazed me was what happened when these same patients made powerful changes in their lives. They began sleeping better. They began saying no. They left unhealthy jobs or relationships. They nourished their bodies. They reconnected to joy. And most importantly, they believed they could heal. The results spoke for themselves.

Quick fixes do not work for chronic diseases

We live in a society that glorifies speed—instant results, instant relief. But chronic diseases don't form overnight, and they don't disappear overnight either. They require a process of deep repair, transformation, and education.

Many patients ask if they should do chemotherapy or radiation. I always tell them the decision is theirs. The LifeBoss program supports you regardless of the path you choose—integrative healing works alongside clinical treatments. But what matters most is *ownership* of your process. When you decide to be in charge, you tap into a strength that no medication can provide.

Rewiring the subconscious mind

I learned early on that true healing must begin in the mind. This is why Hypnocell® was born—to give people access to the language of their cells, to travel deep into the subconscious mind, and communicate healing messages to the body. Why is this important? Because your cells are listening.

Thoughts create chemistry. The subconscious stores not only memories but belief systems that shape your biology. Through hypnosis or consistent meditative practice, we can begin to reprogram the mind, remove fear-based thinking, and install healing-centered beliefs.

For example, people who hold deep-seated resentment or self-blame may unknowingly block their healing potential. But once forgiveness, peace, and clarity are activated, the body's innate regenerative systems begin to turn on again. I've seen patients go from terminal diagnoses to complete remission by transforming their beliefs and emotions.

One of the most powerful things I've learned is that healing is not meant to happen in isolation. If you're going through this journey, you must surround yourself with people who believe in you, speak life into you, and give you energy—not drain it. Cut out toxic relationships and open your heart to genuine support. Positivity is not a luxury—it's part of your prescription.

If you're the one supporting someone with cancer, don't just say "I'm here if you need me." Say: "I'm here *with* you. Let's walk this together." Ask real questions. Listen without judgment. Your presence matters more than your words.

Cancer isn't a death sentence. It's a wake-up call.

Whether you believe this or not yet, cancer can be your opportunity to awaken. It's your body's way of saying something must change. Maybe it's the way you've been eating, the stress you've been carrying, the lifestyle you've been tolerating, or the unresolved traumas you've pushed away for decades.

Let this be your permission to start over.

If you are newly diagnosed, scared, or overwhelmed—know that these feelings are valid. But don't stay there. Use this time to reflect. Learn. Grow. Take radical responsibility for your life. The healing journey is not only about getting rid of disease—it's about becoming the version of yourself you were always meant to be.

And if you are cancer-free, use this book as a preventive guide. Share it. Teach others. Change your habits. Prevention is the most powerful form of medicine.

Your diagnosis is not your identity

Having cancer doesn't mean you *are* cancer. You are a whole, complex, and powerful being—capable of regeneration, resilience, and miracles.

You are not alone.

You are not helpless.

You are not broken.

You are healing. Right now. And this book, this journey, is your first step back to health.

Chapter 2
Can you prevent cancer?

One of the most important insights I've gained through years of working with patients is this: a cancer diagnosis is rarely unexpected by the body. Long before any imaging or biopsy confirms it, the body has already been communicating distress. These early signs often appear six months to two years before the formal diagnosis—sometimes through fatigue, chronic inflammation, digestive issues, emotional instability, sleep disruption, or other subtle symptoms that are too often dismissed or overlooked.

The field of psychoneuroimmunology—which explores the interaction between psychological processes, the nervous system, and immunity—offers compelling evidence that emotional states, chronic stress, trauma, and energetic imbalances can disrupt immune function, alter cellular communication, and create the perfect internal environment for disease to take hold.

This means one vital thing: the process leading to cancer can often be interrupted—or even reversed—when we start listening to the body early enough.

While cancer prevention is still considered a developing field in conventional medicine, rooted in evolving clinical trials and research, it has long been explored in integrative, functional, and lifestyle medicine. In this book, we take a practical and holistic approach, combining what we know from research with natural, proven tools for self-care.

Here, I'll begin by sharing foundational strategies—simple, daily choices that are easy to adopt and can make a significant difference over time. Cancer prevention doesn't have to mean rigid rules or extreme protocols. It's about making conscious, nourishing decisions, one step at a time.

Exercise: movement is medicine

Physical activity is a cornerstone of cancer prevention. In fact, inactivity itself has been identified as a risk factor for several types of cancer, including breast, colon, endometrial, and pancreatic cancers.

Movement improves blood circulation, supports lymphatic detoxification, balances hormones, reduces inflammation, and promotes optimal digestion—all of which are essential in keeping your cells healthy and resilient.

For example, regular movement helps the intestines function more efficiently and can significantly reduce the risk of colorectal cancer by decreasing the time waste stays in the bowel. This minimizes exposure to potentially carcinogenic substances.

Exercise has also been linked to lower levels of estrogen, which can reduce the risk of hormone-related cancers like breast and ovarian. Additionally, staying active helps regulate insulin and insulin-like growth factors (IGFs), which can fuel tumor growth when left unchecked.

How much should you move?

The recommended baseline for general health is at least 150 to 200 minutes of moderate-intensity activity per week, or 30 minutes daily. If you're looking to maximize preventive benefits, aim for 210 to 300 minutes per week, especially if you're at higher risk.

But let me emphasize something: you don't need a gym membership to prevent cancer.

Walking, dancing, hiking, cycling, gardening, and even vigorous housework like sweeping, mopping, and vacuuming all count as physical activity. What matters most is consistency and enjoyment—because if you enjoy your movement, you'll keep doing it.

Here are some tips to make exercise a part of your daily life without the overwhelm:

- Take the stairs instead of the elevator.

- Walk to do errands instead of driving when possible.

- Do gentle stretches or yoga during your lunch break.

- Get off one stop earlier from your bus, metro, or car ride and walk.

- Set a timer to get up and move every hour if you work at a desk.

The key is to think of movement not as a task, but as a gift to your future self—an act of care that builds cellular strength and metabolic resilience.

Yoga: reconnecting mind, body, and energy

Yoga is more than just stretching or flexibility—it is a powerful therapeutic tool. Practicing yoga enhances not only physical function but also mental clarity, emotional regulation, and energetic balance.

Styles like Bikram, Ashtanga, and Vinyasa offer cardiovascular benefits while strengthening muscles and improving detoxification through sweat. But even slower practices like Hatha or Yin yoga offer remarkable benefits by calming the nervous system and improving sleep, digestion, and immune function.

Yoga also teaches Pranayama, or breathwork. These breathing techniques improve oxygenation, activate the vagus nerve, reduce stress hormones, and support the release of metabolic waste. For cancer prevention, this means better cellular respiration, better pH balance, and a stronger defense against chronic inflammation.

Just one hour of yoga per week can:

- Reduce inflammation markers.

- Improve immune surveillance.

- Decrease pain and medication side effects.

- Restore parasympathetic nervous system dominance (your healing state).

- Support emotional resilience and mental calmness.

You don't have to become a yoga expert—just commit to showing up, whether that's once a week at a studio, a short practice at home, or a five-minute morning breathing routine. Every small shift matters.

Healthy lifestyle choices: your daily armor against cancer

When we talk about a healthy lifestyle, we're not simply referring to weight or fitness. We are talking about a collection of intentional, evidence-based habits that form your first line of defense against chronic diseases—especially cancer. Many cancers don't just "happen." They are the result of cumulative damage over time, often influenced by what we consume, how we live, and the environments we expose ourselves to.

Here are eight powerful choices you can begin to make—starting today—to significantly lower your cancer risk and support a resilient body and mind.

1. Avoid tobacco in all forms

Tobacco is still one of the most preventable causes of cancer worldwide. Smoking is directly linked to cancers of the lungs, mouth, throat, larynx, pancreas, bladder, cervix, kidney, and esophagus. Even smokeless tobacco products (such as chewing tobacco and snuff) increase the risk of oral, throat, and pancreatic cancers.

Equally important: second-hand smoke exposure is also a carcinogen. Even brief exposure can cause cell-level damage, especially in children, pregnant women, and the elderly.

If you've smoked in the past or are trying to quit, seek professional support. Programs like Hypnocell® offer an integrative approach using targeted meditations and subconscious rewiring to reduce nicotine cravings, calm anxiety, and restore cellular balance by halting the inhalation of toxic compounds. The moment you stop smoking, your body begins to heal—and that's a biological fact.

2. Protect yourself from the sun

Skin cancer is one of the most common—and also one of the most preventable—cancers. Ultraviolet (UV) radiation from the sun and tanning beds damages the DNA in skin cells, which can lead to mutations and uncontrolled cell growth.

To reduce your risk:

- Avoid direct sun exposure between 10 a.m. and 4 p.m., when UV rays are strongest.

- Always use a broad-spectrum sunscreen (SPF 30 or higher), even on cloudy days.

- Wear protective clothing, sunglasses, and wide-brimmed hats.

- Never use tanning beds or sunlamps—they emit UVA and UVB radiation at levels even more intense than the sun.

Sun protection is a lifelong habit, not a seasonal one.

3. Get vaccinated

Some cancers are triggered by viruses that you can protect yourself against through immunization. Two major vaccines to consider:

- Hepatitis B: Chronic infection can increase the risk of liver cancer. The vaccine is especially recommended for those at higher risk (e.g., healthcare workers or people living in areas where HBV is common).

- Human Papillomavirus (HPV): A major cause of cervical, vaginal, vulvar, penile, anal, and throat cancers. The vaccine is now widely recommended for both boys and girls starting around age 11 or 12.

By preventing the infections that can cause cancer, you cut off the disease at one of its earliest roots.

4. Prioritize routine medical care and screenings

Early detection saves lives. Regular screenings can help identify precancerous conditions or cancer at a stage when it's still treatable.

Speak to your healthcare provider about:

- Pap smears and HPV tests (cervical cancer)

- Mammograms (breast cancer)

- Colonoscopy or stool tests (colorectal cancer)

- PSA test (prostate cancer)

- Skin checks, especially if you have many moles or a family history of melanoma

Age, family history, and risk factors all determine when to start screening—so personalize your approach with your physician.

5. Avoid risky behaviors

Some viruses and bacteria associated with cancer are spread through risky behaviors.

To reduce your risk:

- Practice safe sex (use condoms and limit sexual partners)

- Avoid sharing needles, especially in drug use, tattooing, or piercing

- Be cautious with blood and body fluids, especially in healthcare or caregiving settings

Key cancer-associated viruses include:

- HIV: Linked to Kaposi's sarcoma, lymphoma, and cervical cancer.

- Hepatitis B and C: Major risk factors for liver cancer.

- Epstein-Barr Virus (EBV): Linked to nasopharyngeal carcinoma and certain lymphomas.

- Herpes Simplex Virus: Associated with Kaposi's sarcoma in immunocompromised individuals.

- HPV: A common virus strongly linked to cervical and other genital cancers.

These infections are not just short-term risks—they can have lifelong consequences for cellular health.

6. Be mindful of what you wear, apply, and inhale

Your skin is your largest organ, and it absorbs more than we often realize. Many cosmetics, personal care products, and even clothing contain chemicals classified as Group 1 carcinogens by the WHO, including:

- Formaldehyde

- Coal tar

- Benzene

- Glyphosate (herbicide)

- Phthalates and parabens

- Bleach and chlorine

These substances are commonly found in:

- Shampoos, hair dyes, and conditioners

- Nail polish and remover

- Tampons and sanitary pads

- Non-organic baby clothing and flame-retardant pajamas

- Dry-cleaned clothes, chemically treated towels and sheets

Air pollution is another major source of daily toxin exposure. If you live in a city or near heavy traffic, you may be breathing in ozone, diesel particles, and volatile organic compounds (VOCs) that increase cancer risk. An air purifier at home and plants like aloe vera and peace lilies can help filter indoor air.

7. Choose your food consciously

Every bite you take either fights disease or feeds it. Diet plays a pivotal role in cancer development—and prevention. Unfortunately, many people only review their eating habits after diagnosis.

Here are some Group 1 and 2A carcinogens in food (WHO classification):

- Processed meats (hot dogs, bacon, salami)

- Red meats cooked at high temperatures

- Nitrates and nitrites in preserved foods

- Refined sugar and high-fructose corn syrup

- Glyphosate in non-organic produce

- Fried foods that produce acrylamides (e.g., French fries)

Prevention starts by minimizing these and choosing whole, plant-based, anti-inflammatory foods. Focus on:

- Colorful vegetables and fruits (rich in polyphenols and antioxidants)

- Cruciferous veggies (broccoli, cabbage, kale)

- Omega-3 fats (flaxseeds, wild salmon)

- Turmeric, ginger, and garlic

- Fiber-rich foods that support detox and gut health

Food is information. What you eat tells your cells how to behave.

8. Prioritize deep, restorative sleep

Sleep is not a luxury—it is a fundamental component of immune function, detoxification, cellular repair, and hormonal balance.

Disrupted circadian rhythms and insufficient sleep are associated with:

- Reduced melatonin (a powerful antioxidant with anti-cancer properties)

- Impaired T-cell function and natural killer cell activity

- Elevated cortisol and inflammation

To optimize sleep:

- Maintain a consistent bedtime routine.

- Eliminate screen time at least 1 hour before bed.

- Keep your room cool, dark, and quiet.

- Avoid heavy meals, alcohol, or caffeine in the evening.

- Try deep breathing or Hypnocell® sleep meditations to support mental unwinding.

Your body does most of its repair during deep sleep. Make it count.

Food choices: eating with intention to lower cancer risk

While food alone may not completely eliminate the risk of cancer, decades of research have shown that mindful eating habits can dramatically reduce your chances of developing it. Food is not only fuel—it's information that communicates with your cells. What you put on your plate can either help your body repair and regenerate or fuel chronic inflammation and disease.

Eat a diet rich in plants

Start by filling your plate with a rainbow of fruits and vegetables. These plant-based foods are packed with:

- Fiber to aid detoxification and support gut health

- Vitamins and minerals essential for immune and metabolic function

- Phytochemicals, powerful compounds that protect cells from DNA damage and abnormal growth

Aim for a wide variety of colors—greens, reds, oranges, purples, and whites—because each color provides unique protective compounds. Whole grains, legumes, beans, seeds, and nuts should also be staples in your diet.

Minimize alcohol—or avoid it entirely

Alcohol consumption is a known risk factor for several cancers, including:

- Breast

- Colorectal

- Liver

- Mouth, throat, and esophagus

If you do choose to drink, keep it moderate: up to one drink per day for women and two for men. However, studies show that the safest level of alcohol consumption for cancer prevention is zero.

Limit processed and red meats

Processed meats—like bacon, sausages, ham, and cold cuts—are classified by the World Health Organization as Group 1 carcinogens, meaning there is strong evidence they cause cancer, especially colorectal cancer. Red meats like beef, pork, and lamb are considered Group 2A—probably carcinogenic when consumed in high amounts.

Instead, choose lean proteins like:

- Wild-caught fish (especially fatty fish rich in omega-3)

- Organic eggs

- Lentils, beans, and legumes

- Nuts and seeds

- Plant-based protein sources (e.g., tempeh, quinoa, tofu)

Some patients in my LifeBoss Health program follow the Mediterranean, Paleo, or Keto diets—always tailored to individual health needs. These can be effective when built around anti-inflammatory, nutrient-dense foods.

Don't forget the essentials: calcium and vitamin D

Calcium and Vitamin D are vital in reducing the risk of certain cancers, particularly colorectal and breast cancer. These nutrients:

- Help regulate cell growth

- Support immune system strength

- Assist in maintaining healthy bone structure

Get calcium from leafy greens, almonds, sardines, and fortified plant-based milks. For Vitamin D, a mix of safe sun exposure, fatty fish, and supplementation (if needed) is key.

Avoid highly processed and high-fat foods

Not all fats are bad, but saturated and trans fats—often found in fried foods, baked goods, fast food, and packaged snacks—can contribute to weight gain, inflammation, and metabolic disruption.

Instead, focus on healthy fats, such as:

- Omega-3 fatty acids (from flaxseeds, chia seeds, walnuts, wild salmon)

- Monounsaturated fats (from olive oil, avocado, almonds)

- Polyunsaturated fats (from sunflower seeds, walnuts, soybean oil)

Beets, for example, are a superfood rich in betalains—antioxidant compounds that support liver detoxification and exhibit anticancer, anti-inflammatory, and cell-protective effects.

Phytochemicals: Your body's natural armor

Phytochemicals are naturally occurring compounds found in plants that help the body:

- Neutralize carcinogens

- Slow tumor growth

- Strengthen the immune system

- Balance hormones

- Reduce oxidative stress

Common phytochemical-rich foods include:

- Broccoli (sulforaphane)

- Cranberries (proanthocyanidins)

- Garlic (allicin)

- Carrots (beta-carotene)

- Tomatoes (lycopene)

- Blueberries (anthocyanins)

- Cauliflower, cabbage, and kale (indoles and glucosinolates)

- Grapefruit and citrus fruits (limonoids)

These foods are part of what I call "Nature's Defense System."

Superfoods I recommend for cancer prevention

From my clinical and integrative experience, here are my go-to cancer-fighting foods:

- Broccoli – Rich in sulforaphane, helps flush out carcinogens

- Cranberries – Powerful antioxidants that protect cells

- Garlic – Enhances immune function and detox pathways

- Carrots – Beta-carotene helps slow abnormal cell growth

- Tomatoes – Lycopene helps reduce prostate and breast cancer risk

- Beets – Support liver function and cell detoxification

- Ginger – Anti-inflammatory and promotes digestion

Incorporate these regularly into your meals for a tangible health upgrade.

Ask the right questions—and find the right guidance

If you're unsure what to eat, ask your doctor or a qualified nutritionist. You can ask:

- What foods can help lower my cancer risk?

- What should I avoid if I've had cancer before?

- Which supplements are safe and effective for prevention?

And if your doctor tells you "food doesn't matter"—which unfortunately still happens—get a second opinion from a health professional who understands the connection between nutrition and chronic disease prevention. Your diet matters more than many think.

Final thoughts

This chapter has outlined practical and powerful dietary choices that serve as both prevention and protection. But beyond cancer, these choices improve your energy, mental clarity, digestion, and longevity.

Nutrition is one of the most empowering tools you can use daily. When paired with physical activity, emotional balance, and quality sleep, it creates a body terrain that's far less welcoming to disease.

In the next chapter, we'll explore more healing principles rooted in science and human biology—but remember, change starts with your plate.

Chapter 3

Cancer diagnosis? Now what?

In Chapter One, we touched briefly on how it feels to receive a cancer diagnosis and the immediate steps a person can take. That initial chapter had to introduce the emotional and mental foundation necessary to begin the healing journey, and while it only scratched the surface, it planted an important seed.

Now, in this chapter, we're going deeper. I'm going to share the tools, insights, and real strategies I've witnessed helping many of my patients—people who regained not only their health but also their sense of personal power. These are not abstract ideas. These are practical, real-world strategies that support the mind-body connection and allow you to step into the role of active participant in your recovery.

First and foremost: don't isolate yourself

After a cancer diagnosis, one of the worst things you can do is isolate yourself emotionally or socially. Many people feel shocked, scared, ashamed, or overwhelmed. Some withdraw, thinking they need to "process it alone." But isolation can create a toxic emotional environment—one that fuels fear and weakens your inner strength.

Instead, seek connection. Find support through friends, family, spiritual communities, coaches, or healing groups. Even if you feel like no one understands, I promise—many people do. And you need that emotional support as much as you need medical guidance.

This doesn't mean you have to share your entire journey with everyone. But having a trusted circle who listens, uplifts, and believes in your strength makes a world of difference.

Regaining control after a diagnosis

One of the hardest parts of being diagnosed with cancer is the feeling of losing control. The system often tells you:

- What to do

- When to do it

- What not to question

Suddenly, you become a patient, not a person. The fear grows, and the belief in your own healing power shrinks.

Many of my patients have described this moment as "handing over the keys" to someone else—usually the doctors, the hospital, or the treatment protocol. And while this may feel necessary in the beginning, staying in that passive role can disempower your entire system—mentally, emotionally, and energetically.

Let me be very clear: I'm not telling you to reject conventional medicine. But I am asking you to stay in the driver's seat of your own life. The greatest healing outcomes happen when you are active in your recovery, when you believe in your body's capacity to heal, and when you trust your intuition.

What about alternative and complementary therapies?

Over the past decade, more people around the world have begun to explore integrative approaches to cancer treatment—ones that combine the best of both worlds: medical science and holistic healing.

This movement toward complementary therapies—such as nutritional healing, meditation, hypnotherapy, herbal medicine, breathwork, detoxification, and emotional release work—gives patients a new tool: agency.

With conventional treatment, you're often asked to "trust the system"—to take a pill, follow a protocol, and wait. This can feel passive, rigid, or overwhelming.

With complementary therapies, you start participating actively in your healing. You begin asking questions like:

- What is my body trying to tell me?

- What emotional or energetic root might be involved?

- How can I support my immune system, metabolism, or cellular regeneration?

- What can I do today to feel stronger, lighter, more hopeful?

This is the kind of inquiry that starts to awaken the healing intelligence already present in your body.

But should I choose one or the other?

Here's the truth: you don't have to choose. You can combine them.

When you incorporate safe and evidence-based alternative therapies alongside medical treatments (with your doctor's awareness and consent), you create a more supportive, whole-person approach.

Many of my patients have told me that working with the LifeBoss Health and using tools like Hypnocell®—while also undergoing chemotherapy, surgery, or radiation—allowed them to:

- Recover faster

- Feel more grounded and emotionally stable

- Experience less side effects

- Reclaim a sense of purpose and spiritual connection

This is the power of integrative healing. It doesn't ask you to reject one system in favor of another. It asks you to stay conscious of what serves your body and mind at every step.

If you're under medical treatment now...

If you are currently going through chemotherapy, immunotherapy, or radiation, always speak with your doctor before adding new treatments, even if they're natural. You want to make sure there are no interactions or contraindications.

But if you are between treatments, not yet under medical care, or in remission and rebuilding, then this is the perfect moment to explore and implement the tools this book offers. You are not powerless. You are not at the mercy of a disease. You are more than a diagnosis.

Become a clinical detective of your own life

I often say that healing is like becoming a detective—you investigate not just your disease, but your lifestyle, emotions, habits, beliefs, and relationships. You uncover what your body is trying to tell you through this diagnosis.

This new mindset changes everything. Suddenly, you stop seeing cancer as the enemy and begin seeing it as a messenger. That doesn't make it easy, but it does make it meaningful.

Receiving a cancer diagnosis is often described as one of life's most profound emotional earthquakes. In the space of a single sentence — "You have cancer" — the world stops spinning the way it used to. The air grows heavier, sounds become muffled, and time slows down. That moment divides life into a "before" and an "after," and no matter who you are or what your story has been, everything suddenly feels uncertain.

The first emotion is often shock. Even if the possibility had been mentioned or feared, there is still something surreal and disorienting about hearing it out loud. Shock is the body's way of protecting the mind — a brief pause before the flood of reality pours in. This is when many describe feeling like they're floating above their body, watching the scene unfold from a distance. It's not denial. It's the nervous system trying to find its footing.

Then comes fear — raw, primal, and all-consuming. Fear of pain. Fear of suffering. Fear of change. Fear of loss — not just of life, but of identity, of control, of dreams, of future plans, of who you believed you were. The fear can be so vast it doesn't even have a name, just a heaviness in the chest and a tremble in the bones.

For many, fear is followed by grief. Grief not only for the potential loss of life but for the loss of normalcy. There's mourning for routines, relationships, roles, and even one's own body. You might grieve the idea of growing old, watching your children grow, or the simple pleasures of everyday life that now feel distant or threatened. This grief is quiet, internal, and often unspoken — but it is very r eal.

Anger often finds its way into the heart too. "Why me?" "What did I do to deserve this?" It's a thunderous, righteous rage at the unfairness of it all — the randomness, the cruelty, the disruption. Anger is not a weakness. It is a powerful, natural reaction to helplessness, and when understood, it can fuel the will to fight.

Then there is guilt — a tricky, insidious emotion. Some blame themselves for lifestyle choices, past decisions, or not catching it earlier. Others feel guilty for burdening their loved ones, for being "weak," or for needing help. Guilt rarely has logic behind it, but it clings to the soul and must be gently unwrapped with compassion.

In the midst of this emotional storm, one of the most difficult companions is loneliness. Even surrounded by loved ones, people often describe feeling alone in their experience — as if no one can truly understand the internal chaos. This loneliness is not from lack of support but from the depth of the journey, which can feel isolating.

But eventually, and almost miraculously, other emotions begin to rise. Hope shows up — sometimes quietly, in the voice of a doctor, the words of a survivor, or in the gentle embrace of a friend. Gratitude finds its way in — not because of the illness, but despite it. Gratitude for the present moment, for small wins, for laughter, for breath, for another sunrise.

And above all, there is resilience. That inner strength we never knew we had. The quiet decision to try, to show up, to keep going. Resilience doesn't mean ignoring the fear or sadness — it means holding them in one hand and courage in the other.

Every patient who receives a cancer diagnosis rides this emotional rollercoaster in their own way. But at the core, these feelings — the fear, the grief, the strength, the hope — are deeply human and universally shared. You are not broken for feeling them. You are not alone in them. You are not weak.

Surfing the wave of uncertainty: recommendations for the newly diagnosed

A cancer diagnosis is a tidal wave — sudden, overwhelming, and often disorienting. It crashes through your mind, pulling you into a current of fear, confusion, and doubt. But even the strongest waves can be surfed. You don't need to fight the ocean — you need to learn to ride it, one breath, one decision, one moment at a time.

Here are recommendations to help you navigate the early days after your diagnosis — a time that is often the most emotionally intense, but also a powerful turning point:

1. Breathe First, Decide Later

Give yourself space. You don't have to make every decision today. Take a few deep breaths — literally. This is not just a metaphor; slowing your breath activates your parasympathetic nervous system and helps reduce panic. Ground yourself before taking any action.

2. Get the facts, not the fears

The internet is full of horror stories. Avoid going down rabbit holes that leave you more confused and scared. Instead, write down your questions and bring them to your oncologist or a trusted integrative physician. Ask for clarity on your specific diagnosis: the type of cancer, its stage, the treatment options, and the prognosis for your case — not for statistics.

3. Build Your Circle

Choose who you want in your support circle. Some people will comfort you, others will drain you. Don't feel guilty for setting boundaries. You're allowed to say, "I need quiet," or "I'll share when I'm ready." Choose to be surrounded by those who bring calm, not chaos.

4. Take notes or bring a second set of ears

In appointments, take notes or bring a loved one who can help you remember what was said. Your emotions might make it hard to absorb everything at once. It's okay to ask doctors to repeat information or explain it in simpler terms.

5. Honor your emotions

You don't have to be strong every minute. Cry if you need to. Scream if you must. Laugh if you feel like it. Emotions will move through you like waves — none are wrong. Acknowledge them instead of fighting them. Suppressing fear or sadness only delays healing.

6. Ask for a timeline, then live outside it

Some patients obsess over timelines: "How long do I have?" or "When will this end?" Ask your doctors about expectations, but then give yourself permission to live beyond the numbers. No one is a statistic. Healing is unpredictable — and that includes miracles, too.

7. Consider a second opinion

Even the best doctors can have different perspectives. Getting a second opinion is not a betrayal — it's wise. It can offer reassurance, additional options, or new approaches, especially if you're considering integrative or regenerative treatments.

8. Begin a health journal

Writing is a powerful tool for healing. Document your thoughts, symptoms, progress, and questions. This is not just a medical record — it's an emotional compass. Journaling helps you notice patterns, track improvements, and reflect on how far you've come.

9. Create a healing space

Whether it's a quiet corner at home or a garden, claim a space that feels peaceful. Surround it with things that nourish your soul: candles, music, books, plants, prayer items, or photographs. Let this become your safe haven when the world feels too loud.

10. Feed your body with care

Nutrition plays a vital role in supporting your immune system and metabolism. Ask your doctor or a cancer nutritionist for guidance. Opt for whole, anti-inflammatory foods, hydration, and possibly supplements — but never self-prescribe. Get professional support to build a plan for your unique needs.

11. Learn to meditate or practice mindfulness

Even five minutes a day of mindfulness, guided breathing, or meditation can help lower cortisol, increase clarity, and boost emotional resilience. Your mind is not your enemy. It can become your most powerful healing ally when gently trained.

12. Explore complementary therapies

From acupuncture and massage to Hypnocell®, hypnosis, or sound therapy — many patients find relief, empowerment, and inner healing through complementary approaches. These methods help balance the emotional and energetic bodies, which are deeply affected by cancer.

13. Let Go of the idea of "going back to normal"

You are transforming — not breaking. You may not go back to how things were before, but you can move toward something even stronger, wiser, and more aligned. This is not about erasing the fear. It's about building your new life with intention and courage.

14. Don't wait to live

Your life does not pause just because you are facing cancer. Continue to love, laugh, explore, plan, and even dream. Yes, some days will be harder. But others will surprise you with beauty. Keep your eyes open for those days. They are sacred.

Reclaiming the power within: Taking ownership of your healing journey

When someone hears the word cancer, they often feel their body is no longer their own. Suddenly, life is split between before the diagnosis and after. Doctors, appointments, scans, and protocols take center stage, and the person at the center of it all — you — may begin to feel more like a passive recipient than an active participant in your own healing.

This is natural. Our medical systems are structured around urgency and authority. We are trained to trust professionals (and we should — they save lives), but sometimes, in the process, we abandon our own inner compass.

It is time to reclaim that compass.

You Are not powerless — You are a co-creator

Doctors bring knowledge, science, and incredible tools. But you bring something equally powerful: your beliefs, your intuition, your choices, and your will to live. Healing is not something done to you — it is a process you participate in.

Even the most effective treatments work best when the patient is fully involved — physically, mentally, emotionally, and spiritually. When you shift from "What will the doctors do for me?" to "What can I do for my body and mind to support this process?", you move from fear to freedom.

Why patients often feel they have no control

The modern medical model is built around diagnosis, protocol, and compliance. While structure is important, it can make patients feel like passengers. You might fear that if you deviate from the plan, or add your own ideas, you'll "mess it up" or be judged. This creates a false belief: "If I don't follow blindly, I'll fail."

But true healing doesn't come from blind obedience — it comes from conscious collaboration.

You are not just a case or a number. You are a whole person, and your voice matters. Your healing depends not just on what is done to you, but on how connected you feel to your body, your treatment, and your life.

How to regain trust in your body and mind

1. Learn with curiosity, not panicResearch holistic or integrative approaches from a place of calm curiosity, not fear or urgency. Knowledge empowers you when it's grounded in intention, not

desperation.

2. Ask yourself: What feels right?Listen to your intuition. If a treatment feels off, explore why. If you feel called toward meditation, breathwork, fasting, clean nutrition, or energy healing — investigate it. The body often whispers what it needs.

3. Integrate, don't replaceTaking control doesn't mean rejecting conventional medicine. It means adding layers of support that honor your inner wisdom. Your oncologist treats the disease; you treat the terrain — your mind, emotions, beliefs, and energy field.

4. Build a healing routine you controlCreate daily rituals that remind you of your power:

   ◦ A healing affirmation every morning.

   ◦ A 5-minute visualization of healthy cells.

   ◦ Choosing foods that support regeneration.

   ◦ Time in nature or quiet.

   ◦ Self-hypnosis or meditations from Hypnocell®.These are your decisions, not prescriptions. That shift makes all the difference.

5. Choose language that empowersSay, "I'm healing" not "I'm sick."Say, "I'm partnering with my doctors" not "They are saving me."Say, "I trust my body's wisdom" not "My body betrayed me."Words rewire your reality.

6. Let go of the need for full controlYou can't control every outcome — but you can control your environment, your attitude, your breath, your thoughts. Control is not power. Presence is. Alignment is. Trust is. Let those guide you.

Healing is an inside-out process

The most profound healing I've witnessed in my patients did not come from a magic pill or procedure. It came when they stopped delegating their power and began reconnecting with their purpose, their bodies, and their inner voice.

It came when they asked: What is this disease trying to teach me? And then answered: I am stronger than I thought. I still have so much life to live. I choose to heal.

This is not wishful thinking. It's conscious participation in your recovery. It is choosing faith over fear, action over passivity, self-love over helplessness.

You are not "just a patient." You are the captain of your healing journey. Doctors will walk beside you — but you must take the first step within.

Cancer may have entered your life, but it does not get to define your story. You are not just a patient — you are a person: a soul, a fighter, a dreamer, a creator of your own healing path.

Surf the wave. You are not alone. And you are stronger than you ever imagined.

You are awakening.

Because within the breakdown, there is the possibility of breakthrough. And within the shaking ground of diagnosis, there is also the foundation for healing — not just of the body, but of the heart, the soul, and the story you are still writing.

In the next section, we'll explore how to build your personal healing plan using the power of the subconscious mind, nutrition, cellular regeneration, and energetic alignment. But before we get there, I want you to absorb this one truth:

You are not broken. You are awakening.

Chapter 4

We are what we eat

This is not just a metaphor—it's a physiological reality. Everything you put into your body either contributes to your healing or feeds disease. Every bite is a message to your cells, and those messages accumulate over time, creating either balance or dysfunction.

If you consistently ingest unhealthy foods—laden with refined sugars, processed ingredients, artificial chemicals, and inflammatory oils—your body will struggle. The nutrients your cells rely on will be scarce, and toxins will accumulate. Over time, your metabolism will slow, your immune system will weaken, and your natural detox systems—like your liver and digestive tract—will be overwhelmed.

On the other hand, if you choose a vibrant, healing diet rich in vitamins, minerals, enzymes, antioxidants, and fiber, you give your body the best chance to restore equilibrium. Your energy improves. Your digestion becomes mor e efficient. Your mind feels sharper. Your cells can repair, replicate, and rejuvenate. You empower your body to heal.

Food is cancer's greatest enemy—never forget that. Real food is real medicine.

Your body wants to heal—give it what it needs

You have the power to deliver natural medicine to your body every single day, simply through the food you choose. Take this moment in your life as an opportunity to look closely and consciously at what you're eating.

Remember the anti-cancer foods I mentioned in earlier chapters? These are not just preventive—they're therapeutic. They are powerful allies during cancer treatment and recovery.

At the beginning of my LifeBoss® program, I often recommend a 21-day detox protocol. This is a gentle but targeted reset that focuses on:

- Cleansing the digestive system

- Strengthening the immune system

- Starving cancer cells of their preferred fuel

Cancer feeds on sugar

Let me be direct: cancer cells thrive on sugar. Not just table sugar—but anything that breaks down into glucose quickly. That includes white bread, pasta, refined grains, fruit juices, pastries, and even so-called "natural" sweeteners like honey, agave, and syrups.

I've met countless patients who were offered sugary snacks, juices, or biscuits after chemotherapy or radiation sessions. This horrifies me. How can we expect healing from a disease that thrives on sugar if we're actively feeding it after toxic treatments?

Studies have shown that cancer cells in vitro divide faster and more aggressively in sugar-rich environments. Sugar isn't just a treat—it's a trigger.

That's why one of the first and non-negotiable dietary changes in my program is the complete elimination of added sugars and simple carbohydrates—cold turkey. We also remove artificial sweeteners, which can be equally harmful. Instead, I guide patients into a therapeutic ketogenic, vegetarian or vegan diet, at least during the detox and immune-reset phase.

What to eat instead

Focus on anti-inflammatory, antioxidant-rich, and immune-boosting foods, such as
:

- Leafy greens (spinach, kale, arugula)

- Cruciferous vegetables (broccoli, cauliflower, cabbage)

- Nuts and seeds (chia, pumpkin, sunflower, flax)

- Spices and herbs (turmeric, ginger, garlic, rosemary)

- Low-glycemic fruits (berries, green apples)

- Fermented foods (sauerkraut, kimchi, kefir—if dairy is tolerated)

I invite you to visit my website, and download my free guide to immune-boosting herbs and spices.

How your diet evolves over time

When you start your self-healing journey, your focus should be on detoxification and immune optimization. Once your body starts to stabilize and regain strength, we move into a maintenance phase, where your nutrition plan becomes your long-term lifestyle.

This transformation takes time—it doesn't happen in a week. It's a process of cellular retraining and microbiome restoration, and it often takes several months of consistency to feel the full effects. But trust me, it is worth it.

What about meat?

During the detox phase, I recommend avoiding all red and processed meats. Red meat has been classified as probably carcinogenic to humans (Group 2A), and processed meats (like bacon, sausages, and deli meats) are classified as Group 1 carcinogens—in the same group as tobacco.

Some of my patients decide to eliminate red meat completely and never go back. Others choose to reintroduce it after one or two years. If you do decide to eat meat again, choose organic, grass-fed, hormone-free options in very limited quantities.

The key is to listen to your body. During cancer recovery, your digestive system is delicate. Protein should come from fish, plant sources, or lean poultry—cooked lightly and without added toxins.

A word about the Western diet

The typical Western diet—high in sugar, low in fiber, overloaded with processed food—is a major contributor to chronic diseases like heart disease, diabetes, obesity, and cancer.

In fact, I believe that we're nutritionally starving in a land of abundance. We eat a lot, but we're constantly undernourished.

One of my greatest influences, the late Dr. John Richardson, shared a simple yet powerful formula that I still use with my patients today:

From the Vegetable Kingdom: Eat everything edible for which you have no intolerance. Consume the whole plant whenever possible. Raw is ideal, but if cooking is necessary, do so lightly and naturally.

From the Animal Kingdom: Eat only skinless poultry and fresh fish. Avoid animal fats. Use natural oils like olive or avocado oil. No beef, pork, bacon, dairy, or highly processed animal products.

Vitamin B15: An unsung ally?

I'd also like to share with you an often-overlooked nutrient: Vitamin B15 (pangamic acid). Although it's not approved for therapeutic use in the U.S., it's been widely studied and used in countries like Russia, Japan, Germany, and Spain.

What makes B15 fascinating is its ability to:

- Improve oxygen utilization in the body

- Support detoxification

- Inhibit cancer cell survival (since cancer cells hate oxygen)

B15 works by enhancing cellular respiration and reducing lactic acid buildup. Since cancer cells rely on fermentation to produce energy in the absence of oxygen (a process called the Warburg effect), improving oxygen metabolism challenges their survival mechanisms.

Natural sources of pangamic acid include:

- Apricot seeds

- Pumpkin and sunflower seeds

- Brown rice

- Cantaloupes

- Watermelon

In supplement form, you may find it labeled as calcium pangamate or dimethylglycine (DMG).

Note: Always consult with your healthcare provider before introducing new supplements, especially if you're undergoing medical treatment.

In summary: your healing begins at the table

What you eat matters more than most people realize. Food is not just fuel. It is information for your cells, medicine for your tissues, and a blueprint for your vitality.

Start where you are. Remove what's toxic. Replenish what's missing. Listen to your body. And most importantly—be consistent.

Your next meal can be a step toward healing.Make it count.

Let's talk about sugar: fuel for cancer

When it comes to cancer and nutrition, few topics are as critical—and as misunderstood—as sugar.

To start, it's important to understand the two main types of sugar we encounter in food:

1. Natural sugars – Found in whole foods like fruits, vegetables, dairy, and honey.

2. Added sugars – Sugars added during processing or preparation, such as those in sodas, baked goods, candy, sauces, energy bars, and even salad dressings.

Both types ultimately break down into glucose in the body, and cancer cells are voracious consumers of glucose. Whether it's a spoonful of honey or corn syrup in packaged snacks, the body does not discriminate. Sugar is sugar—and cancer cells love it.

The Warburg effect: why cancer cells love sugar?

This relationship between sugar and cancer was first described by Dr. Otto Warburg, a German medical doctor and Nobel laureate, in the 1920s. He discovered that cancer cells metabolize glucose differently than healthy cells—a phenomenon now known as the Warburg Effect.

Whereas healthy cells generate energy mainly through aerobic respiration (using oxygen), cancer cells rely heavily on anaerobic glycolysis, a process that ferments glucose for energy—even when oxygen is available. This method is less efficient but much faster, allowing cancer cells to grow and divide rapidly.

Here's what makes it more alarming:

- Cancer cells consume up to 50 times more glucose than normal cells.

- They also have up to 3 times more insulin receptors, which makes them more efficient at drawing glucose from the bloodstream.

This means that every sugary bite or sip you take could be feeding the disease.

Why you must drastically reduce sugar intake?

This isn't just theory. Decades of research support the connection between high sugar consumption and increased cancer risk, growth, and metastasis.

- A 2015 study by MD Anderson Cancer Center found that high sugar intake was linked to an increased risk of breast cancer and its spread to the lungs.

- In 2012, Graham et al. demonstrated that glucose withdrawal impaired the survival of metabolically altered tumor cells. Their research showed that certain tumors are highly sensitive to metabolic restriction.

- Numerous studies have since confirmed that low-glycemic and ketogenic diets, combined with intermittent fasting, can help starve cancer cells, slow their growth, and improve patient outcomes.

Why a ketogenic and low-glycemic diet works?

Cancer cells depend on glucose for survival and proliferation. By depriving them of their main fuel source, you disrupt their ability to grow. A low-carbohydrate, high-fat, moderate-protein diet, such as the ketogenic diet, is designed to:

1. Reduce blood glucose levels

2. Lower insulin and insulin-like growth factors

3. Decrease systemic inflammation

4. Increase ketone production, which cancer cells cannot use efficiently for energy

When paired with intermittent fasting, these effects are amplified. Fasting induces autophagy, a natural cellular cleaning process that removes damaged cells and can suppress cancer development.

The power of plants: why a vegetarian or vegan diet can improve outcomes in cancer patients

Nutrition is one of the most accessible and impactful tools a cancer patient has to support their body. While conventional treatment targets the disease, your daily food choices shape the environment in which your cells live, heal, or decay. Among the most transformative shifts a cancer patient can make is adopting a plant-based, vegetarian, or vegan diet.

This isn't a fad. It's a life-affirming approach supported by a growing body of research — and by thousands of patients who have seen firsthand how changing what's on their plate can change the way they feel, respond to treatment, and recover.

Cancer thrives in certain environments — and you can change that

Cancer cells are influenced by the terrain in which they exist: your body's pH, inflammation levels, hormone activity, blood sugar stability, and immune function. These internal conditions are profoundly impacted by food. Unlike processed, high-fat, or animal-heavy diets, plant-based diets support the body's natural healing terrain.

Here's how:

1. Plants fight inflammation — the root of many cancers

Chronic inflammation creates an environment conducive to cancer growth and spread. Animal products (especially processed meats, red meats, and high-fat dairy) have been linked to increased inflammatory markers like C-reactive protein (CRP).

On the other hand, a vegetarian or vegan diet — rich in fruits, vegetables, legumes, nuts, seeds, and whole grains — is loaded with phytonutrients and antioxidants that reduce inflammation, protect DNA, and improve immune regulation.

Key anti-inflammatory compounds include:

- Quercetin (onions, apples)

- Curcumin (turmeric)

- Sulforaphane (broccoli sprouts)

- Resveratrol (grapes, berries)

- Polyphenols (green tea, dark chocolate, berries)

These compounds actively block tumor growth pathways, enhance detoxification, and support healthy gene expression.

2. Fiber supports detoxification and gut health

Animal products contain no fiber — none. A vegan diet, by contrast, is naturally high in soluble and insoluble fiber, which is essential for:

- Maintaining healthy digestion

- Removing toxins and excess hormones (especially estrogen, linked to breast and ovarian cancers)

- Supporting a healthy microbiome (which regulates immunity and inflammation)

A thriving gut microbiome improves treatment tolerance, reduces infection risk, and modulates cancer-fighting immune cells like NK cells and T-cells.

3. Plant-based diets lower IGF-1, a hormone that promotes cancer growth

Insulin-like growth factor 1 (IGF-1) is a hormone involved in cell proliferation. High levels of IGF-1 — common in high-protein, animal-heavy diets — have been linked to increased risk of prostate, breast, and colon cancers.

Studies show that a plant-based diet lowers IGF-1 levels significantly, reducing the hormonal signal for tumor growth. In other words, by removing animal protein and increasing plant foods, patients can starve the signals that feed cancer.

4. Weight and blood sugar are stabilized

Obesity and insulin resistance are risk factors for many types of cancer, as they contribute to chronic inflammation, hormonal imbalance, and oxidative stress. Plant-based diets are naturally lower in calories, rich in complex carbohydrates, and help maintain steady glucose and insulin levels.

Several clinical trials, including studies from Dean Ornish and Dr. Neal Barnard, show that vegan diets can:

- Reverse heart disease

- Stabilize blood sugar

- Promote healthy weight loss

- Improve energy and mood

- And potentially slow cancer progression

5. Phytonutrients promote apoptosis and inhibit angiogenesis

Some plant compounds directly induce apoptosis (programmed death) in cancer cells and inhibit angiogenesis (the creation of blood vessels tumors need to grow). These natural mechanisms are part of why certain foods are called anti-cancer foods.

Notable examples:

- Cruciferous vegetables (broccoli, cabbage): rich in glucosinolates

- Allium vegetables (garlic, leeks): rich in allicin and organosulfur compounds

- Berries: packed with ellagic acid and anthocyanins

- Green tea: EGCG inhibits tumor cell proliferation

These aren't just protective — they are therapeutic.

6. Psychological empowerment

Adopting a vegetarian or vegan diet is more than a nutritional shift — it's a mindset shift. It's a declaration that I am participating in my healing. It gives patients a sense of agency, which helps combat the helplessness that often accompanies a diagnosis.

Patients who change their diets feel more in control, more connected to their bodies, and more proactive in their journey. This mindset can improve quality of life, adherence to treatment, and emotional resilience.

Scientific backing

Numerous studies support these findings:
- The Adventist Health Study found that vegetarians had a significantly lower risk of all cancers compared to non-vegetarians, especially gastrointestinal and female reproductive cancers.

- A 2015 meta-analysis published in the American Journal of Clinical Nutrition found that vegans had a 15% lower risk of developing cancer.

- The Ornish Lifestyle Medicine Program, which includes a low-fat vegan diet, demonstrated a reversal of early-stage prostate cancer in some patients.

The bottom line: plant foods heal

There is no magic bullet. But every plate, every bite, and every choice becomes part of the healing terrain. A vegetarian or vegan diet is not a replacement for medical treatment — it is a powerful complement that supports the body's ability to regenerate, detoxify, and thrive.

This is about turning your kitchen into a pharmacy, and your meals into medicine.

Choose foods that fight for you. Choose habits that heal. Choose to believe that your body — when nourished, loved, and supported — knows how to find its way back to balance.

Key takeaways about sugar and cancer

Let's summarize what we know so far:

1. Tumor cells need glucose to survive and thrive.

2. Carbohydrate restriction reduces blood glucose and insulin, effectively depriving cancer cells of their main fuel.

3. A ketogenic diet and intermittent fasting can regulate metabolic imbalances seen in advanced cancer patients.

4. Reducing carbohydrate intake reduces inflammation, another major contributor to cancer growth and progression.

5. Added sugars (sucrose, high-fructose corn syrup, maltodextrin) and high-glycemic carbohydrates (white bread, pasta, cereals) should be avoided entirely.

6. Even natural sugars (fruit juices, honey, dried fruit) can spike glucose and should be strictly limited during cancer therapy.

A holistic approach to sugar detox

At the beginning of my LifeBoss® cancer program, we always begin with a deep sugar detox as part of the 21-day metabolic reset. This includes:

- Eliminating all forms of added sugar

- Avoiding high-glycemic carbohydrates

- Incorporating healthy fats and antioxidant-rich vegetables

- Integrating herbal support to manage cravings and inflammation

Remember: you are not just dieting—you are starving the disease.

Fasting: a powerful ally in cancer prevention and recovery

Fasting is the voluntary abstention from food—and sometimes drinks—for a specific period of time. While water is typically allowed (and encouraged), all sources of calories are restricted. This ancient practice has been part of religious rituals, healing traditions, and survival periods long before the rise of modern agriculture.

From a clinical perspective, fasting is now recognized as one of the most powerful tools for detoxification, cellular repair, and metabolic balance. In recent years, it has gained substantial scientific backing as an effective complementary therapy in cancer prevention and support.

Why fasting works?

Each time we eat, especially high-glycemic or sugary foods, we stimulate the production of insulin, a hormone that not only manages blood sugar but also influences inflammation, fat storage, and cellular growth—including cancer cell proliferation. By abstaining from food, we allow the body to:

- Enter a deep state of cellular repair (autophagy)

- Reduce insulin levels and inflammation

- Shift from glucose to fat as the main energy source (ketosis)

- Eliminate damaged cells and metabolic waste products

- Strengthen the immune system

Fasting gives your body time to complete digestive processes, clear metabolic byproducts, and switch on healing pathways that are otherwise suppressed in a constantly fed state.

How long should you fast?

There are many fasting protocols, but for general cancer prevention and immune system support, I recommend a gentle intermittent fasting approach:

- Fast for 12–14 hours daily, ideally finishing your last meal by 5:00 PM.

- Only drink pure water (or herbal tea, if necessary) until your first meal the next morning, between 5:00–8:00 AM.

- During eating hours, choose clean, nutrient-dense foods such as vegetables, healthy fats, and high-quality protein.

This method, also known as Time-Restricted Eating (TRE), allows the digestive system and metabolism to reset daily, without the stress of long fasting periods.

Note: Some patients gradually extend their fast to 16 or even 18 hours as they adapt. Others opt for supervised longer fasts (24-72 hours) occasionally under professional guidance, especially in detox or early cancer support protocols.

Fasting and "sticky blood": what Chinese Medicine teaches us

In Traditional Chinese Medicine (TCM), cancer risk has long been associated with "sticky blood", a condition where the blood becomes more viscous or prone to clotting. This concept aligns closely with what modern medicine identifies as hypercoagulation or elevated platelet activity—both of which are common in cancer patients.

How this relates to cancer?

- Platelets, the blood components responsible for clotting, can be hijacked by cancer cells.

- Some tumors stimulate platelet production to form a protective shield around themselves, hiding from immune cells and reducing the effectiveness of chemotherapy.

- These "cloaked" cancer cells can also travel through the bloodstream more easily, increasing the risk of metastasis.

- Fibrin, a sticky protein involved in clot formation, becomes elevated during this process. High fibrinogen levels are linked to cancer progression and poorer outcomes.

Sugar, clotting, and the fibrin connection

Here's where fasting becomes essential again. High glucose intake contributes to elevated fibrinogen levels, making the blood stickier and promoting clotting and tumor protection.

- Sugary diets = More fibrinogen → More fibrin → Greater cancer cell protection

- Fasting + low-carb diet = Reduced fibrin production → Less cancer spread

Fasting and cutting sugar go hand in hand. When you remove sugars from your diet and adopt a fasting protocol, you disrupt one of the key survival mechanisms of tumors.

Final thoughts

Fasting isn't starvation—it's strategic rest for your cells. It's an opportunity to break the toxic cycle of overeating, poor metabolism, and cancer-promoting inflammation.

If you are starting the LifeBoss® cancer program, fasting is one of the foundational steps we use to:

- Detoxify the body

- Starve cancer cells of sugar

- Restore cellular intelligence

- Support long-term healing

Start small. Stay consistent. And always work with your physician or integrative care provider when adjusting your dietary habits—especially if you are on medication or undergoing active cancer treatment.

Supplements that work

While nutrition should always come first, diet alone is often not enough, especially when recovering from illness, restoring balance, or detoxifying the body. Modern lifestyles, environmental toxins, poor soil quality, and chronic stress all contribute to nutritional deficiencies—even in those trying to eat well.

If you're starting your healing journey after cancer diagnosis or prevention, it's important to be honest with yourself: even if you begin eating a perfect diet today, your body may take weeks or months to recover from years of suboptimal nutrient intake. That's why, at the beginning of any integrative program, I recommend targeted supplementation to provide an immediate boost of essential nutrients, antioxidants, and metabolic support.

Below are the key supplements I've found most effective in both prevention and support for people dealing with chronic conditions—including cancer.

Berberine

Berberine is a bioactive compound found in several plants, especially the Berberis shrub. It has shown potent anti-inflammatory, anti-microbial, anti-diabetic, and anti-cancer effects, and also supports gut health and metabolic function.

Key benefits:

- Lowers blood sugar levels and insulin resistance

- Reduces systemic inflammation

- Promotes healthy fat metabolism

- Acts as an antiviral and antimicrobial

- Improves intestinal barrier function (especially after chemotherapy)

- Prolongs retention of chemotherapy drugs in cancer cells by acting as a calcium channel blocker—this helps cytotoxic agents remain longer inside dividing cancer cells, enhancing treatment efficacy.

Bonus: Berberine also promotes healing of leaky gut, a common side effect of chemotherapy and immune dysfunction.

Probiotics & prebiotics

Your gut is your second brain—and it's central to immune health. Probiotics are live beneficial microorganisms, while prebiotics are the fibers and nutrients that feed them.

Recommendations:

- Use a broad-spectrum probiotic with at least 100 billion CFUs daily for 2–3 months.

- Look for strains like Lactobacillus and Bifidobacterium.

- Pair them with prebiotic fibers like inulin, chicory root, or resistant starches.

Benefits include:

- Better digestion and nutrient absorption

- Reduced inflammation

- Enhanced immune surveillance

- Improved blood sugar regulation

Turmeric / curcumin

Turmeric contains the active compound curcumin, a powerful antioxidant, anti-inflammatory, and anti-cancer agent used for centuries in Ayurvedic medicine.

Effects on cancer:

- Inhibits cancer cell growth and replication

- Promotes apoptosis (natural cancer cell death)

- Enhances the effectiveness of chemotherapy

- Reduces side effects from radiation or chemo

- Modulates immune function

Make sure to use curcumin extract with piperine (black pepper) to increase absorption by up to 2000%.

Sleep aid supplements

Sleep is when your body repairs, detoxifies, and regenerates. Poor sleep is a major contributor to inflammation, immune suppression, and tumor progression.

Key ingredients:

- Melatonin (linked to reduced risk of breast and prostate cancer)

- L-theanine (calming)

- Magnesium (muscle relaxation, nerve regulation)

- GABA (natural neurotransmitter for relaxation)

- 5-HTP (precursor to serotonin and melatonin)

A study published in the International Journal of Cancer showed that women who worked night shifts had a *30% higher risk* of breast cancer. Similar patterns are seen with prostate cancer in men.

Not everyone reacts the same to every sleep aid. I recommend testing different combinations until you find what works best for your unique biochemistry.

Black seed oil (Nigella sativa)

Black seed oil—derived from Nigella sativa—has been used for over 2000 years and hailed in traditional medicine as "a cure for everything but death."

Main active compound:

Thymoquinone

Benefits include:

- Antioxidant and anti-inflammatory effects

- Anti-carcinogenic activity (shown effective against prostate, breast, liver, kidney, cervix, and skin cancers)

- Protects healthy tissues from radiation damage

- Regulates immune responses

It's also been shown to reduce tumor size in animal models and improve symptoms of asthma, hypertension, and digestive disorders.

Vitamin C (Ascorbic acid)

Vitamin C is one of the most studied vitamins in cancer research, known for its immune-boosting and antioxidant properties.

Key points:

- Stimulates T-lymphocytes and Natural Killer (NK) cells to attack cancer cells.

- Generates hydrogen peroxide that creates reactive oxygen species (ROS)—selectively toxic to cancer cells but safe for normal cells.

- May help reduce chemo side effects and protect healthy tissue.

Humans do not produce vitamin C endogenously. We must get it from food or supplements.

Recommended dosage:

- For cancer prevention or support: 2000 mg/day (oral)

- FDA baseline recommendations:

    ○ Women: 75 mg/day

    ○ Men: 90 mg/day

    ○ Upper safe limit: 2000 mg/day

Tip: For advanced support, some clinics offer intravenous vitamin C therapy, which reaches higher plasma concentrations than oral supplements.

Chapter 5
Integrative therapies

Intravenous Vitamin C, hyperthermia, oxygenation & mind-body healing

When approaching cancer healing holistically, it's important to integrate conventional treatments with complementary therapies that address not just the disease, but the whole person—body, mind, and energy. Below, I outline some of the most powerful integrative therapies that can enhance recovery, alleviate side effects, and boost the body's natural ability to heal.

Intravenous Vitamin C (IVC)

Intravenous (IV) administration of high-dose vitamin C has demonstrated promising outcomes in cancer support protocols. Unlike oral intake, which is limited by intestinal absorption, IV vitamin C allows plasma concentrations to reach levels that turn this well-known antioxidant into a pro-oxidant.

How it works:

- At high concentrations, vitamin C releases hydrogen peroxide, which produces reactive oxygen species (ROS) around tumor tissue.

- These ROS can damage the DNA and mitochondria of cancer cells, leading to cell death—while leaving healthy cells unharmed.

- It effectively saturates the tumor microenvironment with oxygen, making it hostile for cancer growth.

During IV vitamin C therapy, avoid taking other antioxidants like vitamin E or glutathione concurrently, as they may neutralize the oxidative effects that target cancer cells.

Dosage and safety:

- According to studies published by the National Institutes of Health (NIH), IV vitamin C has been safely administered up to 1.5 grams per kg of body weight per day in cancer patients without kidney disease or kidney stones.

  ○ This equals ~75 grams/day for a 110 lb (50 kg) person.

  ○ Or up to 150 grams/day for a 200 lb (91 kg) person.

- Always seek medical supervision from a licensed practitioner trained in integrative oncology for dosage and monitoring.

Hyperthermia (Heat therapy)

Hyperthermia uses heat to weaken or kill cancer cells and improve the efficacy of other treatments like chemotherapy and radiation. Cancer cells are more sensitive to temperature than healthy cells, and hyperthermia can:

- Increase blood flow to tumors (which improves drug delivery).

- Trigger immune responses by creating a heat shock effect.

- Make cancer cells more vulnerable to radiation.

Application methods:

- Whole-body heat via infrared saunas, steam rooms, or hot water immersion.

- Localized hyperthermia using probes, radiofrequency, ultrasound, or heated blankets applied to tumor sites.

Recommended routine:

- Sauna or steam room 3 times per week.

- 10 minutes per session, alternating between dry and wet heat (e.g., infrared sauna + steam).

- Always hydrate well during and after the session. I recommend warm green tea with ginger to boost detoxification.

Oxygen therapy (Hyperbaric oxygen)

Hyperbaric Oxygen Therapy (HBOT) involves breathing 100% oxygen in a pressurized chamber, allowing oxygen to dissolve into all body fluids—plasma, lymph, spinal fluid—reaching areas where blood flow may be limited.

Why it works:

- Tumors thrive in low-oxygen (hypoxic) environments.

- Increasing tissue oxygenation slows tumor progression and enhances treatment efficacy.

- Hypoxia has also been linked to resistance to chemotherapy and radiation, while oxygen reverses this resistance.

HBOT is used in integrative cancer centers around the world and may be especially useful after radiation or surgical recovery.

Mind-body therapies

The emotional and psychological toll of cancer cannot be overstated. Healing must include the nervous system, emotional regulation, and energy body.

Massage therapy

Massage can:

- Reduce pain, tension, and anxiety

- Improve sleep and circulation

- Provide emotional comfort and relaxation

However, it's essential that the massage therapist is trained to work with cancer patients:

- Avoid areas near surgical scars, tumors, or ports

- Use light pressure, especially for those with low blood counts or fragile skin

- Confirm medical clearance if undergoing active treatment

Meditation & mindfulness

Meditation is a proven tool to regulate the autonomic nervous system and reduce the "fight or flight" response—often overactive in cancer patients.

Benefits:

- Lowers cortisol and stress hormone levels

- Enhances immune function

- Improves emotional regulation and mental clarity

Start with 10–30 minutes daily, focusing on your breath, a mantra, or a peaceful image. Apps and guided meditations can be a great entry point.

Tai Chi & Qi Gong

These gentle movement practices from Chinese medicine combine posture, deep breathing, and mindful movement.

Benefits:

- Improves balance, flexibility, and coordination

- Promotes a calm, centered mind

- Encourages gentle lymphatic movement and detoxification

Always work with a certified instructor, and modify any movements that cause discomfort.

Acupuncture

A cornerstone of Traditional Chinese Medicine, acupuncture uses hair-thin needles inserted into specific meridian points to balance energy (Qi) flow throughout the body.

Benefits:

- Reduces nausea, fatigue, and neuropathy during chemo

- Strengthens the immune system and blood production

- Alleviates anxiety and depression

Studies have shown that acupuncture can help reduce treatment-related side effects and improve overall quality of life for cancer patients.

Ensure the practitioner is licensed and experienced with oncology patients, and always uses sterile, single-use needles.

Final thoughts

These therapies are not meant to replace conventional treatment, but to complement and empower it. They place you at the center of your healing journey—restoring not just your body, but your autonomy, vitality, and spirit.

Healing is a multifactorial process. The more layers you address—physical, emotional, energetic—the more you increase your chances for full recovery and renewal.

Yoga: reconnecting mind, body, and breath

We briefly talked about yoga before, but I need to let you know a bit more about it. Yoga is more than a physical practice—it's a 5,000-year-old philosophy of holistic health that originated in India. Rooted in the integration of body, mind, and spirit, yoga offers a powerful, gentle, and deeply healing tool for those facing cancer and its physical and emotional challenges.

For cancer patients, yoga provides:

- Physical support: Through gentle movements and postures (asanas), yoga helps restore flexibility, strength, and balance—even during or after treatments like surgery, chemotherapy, or radiation.

- Mental clarity: The meditative aspect of yoga promotes calm, reduces anxiety, and improves emotional resilience.

- Breath control (pranayama): Deep, controlled breathing enhances lung function, oxygenation, and nervous system regulation.

- Nervous system healing: Yoga activates the parasympathetic system (rest and digest), counteracting the constant stress response many cancer patients live under.

Clinical benefits of yoga for cancer patients

Numerous studies have shown that yoga:

- Reduces chemotherapy-related nausea and fatigue

- Improves sleep quality

- Relieves pain, joint stiffness, and headaches

- Boosts appetite and digestion

- Supports emotional recovery and body image after surgery or treatment

Patients frequently report that yoga helps them feel more in control, reconnect with their bodies, and develop hope during a difficult journey.

Recommendation: Begin with yoga sessions of 60 minutes, three times per week, incorporating stretching, breathwork, and meditation. Over time, you can increase to 90-minute sessions depending on your energy and comfort level.

Bikram Yoga (Hot Yoga)

Bikram Yoga, a form of hot yoga, can be particularly effective in promoting detoxification, circulation, and flexibility. It includes:

- 26 specific postures

- 2 structured breathing techniques

- Held in a heated room (~105°F / 40°C) to increase sweat and blood flow

This form of yoga encourages compression and stretching of different body regions, helping release deep toxins and improving lymphatic drainage.

Note: If you're new to yoga or recovering from surgery, begin with a gentler form of yoga before transitioning to Bikram. Always consult your physician before starting a hot yoga program.

Aromatherapy: healing through the senses

Aromatherapy is the therapeutic use of essential oils derived from plants and herbs. These oils stimulate olfactory receptors and influence brain pathways tied to mood, emotion, and healing.

How aromatherapy helps:

- Alleviates nausea (especially post-chemotherapy)

- Eases pain and muscle tension

- Induces relaxation and better sleep

- Calms emotional overwhelm and anxiety

Most effective essential oils for cancer patients:

- Lavender – calming, sleep-inducing

- Frankincense – grounding, anti-inflammatory, supportive in grief

- Ginger – anti-nausea, stimulates digestion

- Chamomile – soothing for anxiety and insomnia

- Bergamot – mood-boosting

- Eucalyptus – helps breathing and congestion

- Lemon – detoxifying and energizing

These oils can be:
- Diffused into the air

- Diluted and applied to the skin during massage

- Added to bathwater for calming soaks

Tip: Combine aromatherapy with massage, meditation, or yoga for enhanced effects. Inhale deeply, and allow your body to rest.

Managing the social impact of a cancer diagnosis

A cancer diagnosis doesn't only affect your body—it reshapes your entire social reality. Patients often experience isolation, uncertainty, and a shift in relationships. The emotional weight of the disease, paired with the physical fatigue of treatment, may lead some to withdraw from social circles.

Common social challenges:

- Feeling misunderstood or overwhelmed by others' reactions

- Loss of identity or independence

- Difficulty explaining one's condition or limits

- Fear of being a burden to loved ones

- Stigma or avoidance from others who don't know how to respond

However, this withdrawal is not the solution. Social connection is critical for healing.

Building a supportive social environment:

- Communicate your needs clearly to close friends or family. Let them know what helps and what doesn't.

- Join a cancer support group, either in person or online. These communities provide empathy, shared experiences, and hope.

- Designate a trusted friend or family member to help you filter calls, appointments, and visits when energy is low.

- Don't hesitate to seek professional help—a therapist or counselor experienced in oncology can provide emotional tools to navigate the social changes.

Reminder: It's okay to protect your energy. But it's also okay to let people in. Your vulnerability is not weakness—it's courage.

How can a cancer patient manage the social implications of a cancer diagnosis?

A cancer diagnosis is not just a physical or medical experience—it reverberates through every area of life, especially our relationships. One of the most profound challenges patients face is how to navigate the emotional and social consequences of this new reality.

Start with self-awareness and intention

The first step is to recognize that this journey is not one you should walk alone. Social support is not just comforting—it has been proven to influence recovery, emotional resilience, and even survival rates.

At this point in your life, time becomes more precious—and that often shifts your perspective on who and what really matters. Relationships gain new meaning. It is important to be surrounded by people who uplift you, not drain your energy.

Prioritize family bonds, but stay true to your emotional needs

In most cases, family members will be the closest and most immediate source of support. If you have a healthy, respectful relationship with your family, it's helpful to share your diagnosis with them first and allow them to walk this path with you.

Let them be part of your treatment decisions, your care routines, and your emotional journey—if you're comfortable. When there is open communication, the family can serve as the foundation of strength and continuity during difficult times.

However, not every patient feels close to their family, and that's okay. Some may have strained or distant family ties, while others may be navigating their cancer journey completely alone. In those cases, support can come from friends, neighbors, colleagues, online communities, or cancer support groups.

You do not owe anyone your story before you are ready. Share at your own pace, and only with people you trust.

There's no "right way" to handle social disclosure

Some patients choose to be very open, while others prefer to keep their diagnosis private. Both are valid. The emotional toll of telling others about your condition—fielding their reactions, answering questions, and managing sympathy—can be overwhelming. If you're not ready to share, that's your boundary, and you have every right to protect it.

When and how you communicate about your diagnosis is entirely your decision. You may even find that your feelings about disclosure evolve over time—and that's natural.

Build a circle of empathy and safety

Whether it's a family member, a friend, a therapist, or a support group—having a safe emotional outlet is essential. Cancer can feel isolating, even when you're surrounded by people. Choose connection over isolation, but choose wisely. Invest your limited energy in relationships that give back emotionally.

If you find it hard to connect with others in your immediate circle, I highly recommend seeking:

- Cancer support groups (in-person or online)

- Licensed mental health professionals

- Pastoral or spiritual care

- Mind-body practitioners or wellness coaches

How to manage the spiritual implications of a cancer diagnosis

Cancer is often described as a "spiritual wake-up call." Whether or not you identify as religious or spiritual, a life-threatening illness can challenge your beliefs, stir deep questions about existence, and redefine your sense of purpose.

For some, spirituality provides a sense of peace, meaning, and hope. For others, it may raise doubts or even anger. Both experiences are valid.

Spirituality: a source of strength and peace

Spirituality is not limited to religion. It is about connection—to yourself, to others, to nature, to the universe, or to a higher power. Many patients describe feeling a shift in priorities after a diagnosis, moving away from superficial goals and toward more meaningful pursuits.

Those who rely on spirituality often report:

- Greater emotional stability

- Better treatment compliance

- Lower levels of depression and anxiety

- Improved ability to cope with pain, uncertainty, and fear

- A deeper sense of gratitude and connection

Even patients who weren't previously religious sometimes find themselves exploring spiritual or existential practices during this time.

Spiritual practices that can help:

- Listening to spiritual or meditative music

- Guided meditations or visualizations

- Yoga or Tai Chi

- Mindful breathing exercises

- Reading inspirational or religious texts

- Prayer—alone or with others

- Participating in group rituals, ceremonies, or services

- Journaling your emotions and spiritual reflections

If you're religious, consider speaking with a chaplain or spiritual counselor who can help you explore your faith in the context of healing. Many hospitals have trained spiritual care teams for this purpose.

Remember: You are more than a patient. You are a whole person—mind, body, and spirit. Nurturing your inner life can be just as healing as medical treatment.

Final thoughts before choosing a treatment plan

This chapter was dedicated to the inner dimension of healing—your emotions, relationships, and beliefs. These often-overlooked elements are essential parts of the recovery journey.

After a diagnosis, the next big decision is choosing a treatment plan. Whether you lean toward conventional treatments, alternative approaches, or a combination of both, remember this:

You have the right to be informed, supported, and empowered.

In the next chapter, we'll explore the most common conventional treatment options available, including what to expect, how they work, and how to support your body during each phase.

And as always, everything discussed here should be adapted to your unique situation. If your journey looks different, that's okay. There is no one way to heal—only your way.

Chapter 6

Current cancer treatment options

Receiving a cancer diagnosis is life-altering—it marks a before and after in a person's journey. Yet alongside the fear and confusion, it can also become a powerful opportunity to deepen your understanding of your body and how it heals. While cancer is undeniably a struggle, I want to emphasize that you do not need to feel powerless at any stage. Your attitude, mindset, and ability to stay informed can make a tremendous difference.

I have seen it firsthand: many patients have not only survived cancer but have also emerged stronger and more connected with their bodies, minds, and purpose. Healing comes not just from treatments, but from a profound commitment to oneself.

Let me begin this chapter with a quote that deeply resonated with me, originally written by Martin Wayne in The Townsend Letter for Doctors and Patients, and later cited by Jane McLelland in her remarkable book. It offers clarity on the structure—and challenges—within the medical system:

There are four distinct groups of people involved in making up the medical establishment:

1. Sincere, honest, able investigators who can and have followed revolutionary lines of thought, to the everlasting benefit of mankind.

2. Men just as honest and sincere, but who are or have been enchanted with false concepts and who in a misguided manner would sponsor either

worthless or harmful modalities.

3. Dishonest, incompetent or deceitful individuals who, in seeking self-advantage, would risk or actually cause harm to humanity.

4. Investigators who work for large profit-making corporations who often do not have the wherewithal to object to their work being distorted or shelved for reasons of profit.

This quote illustrates a fundamental truth: not all professionals within the system are the same. And not all treatments or recommendations are made with your best interest at heart. That is why I strongly encourage patients to work with integrative oncologists—doctors who are open to combining conventional cancer treatments with natural and holistic therapies, empowering the patient in their journey.

Understanding your treatment options

In this chapter, we will explore the conventional Western cancer treatments, their intended purpose, and how they might be used in conjunction with alternative or integrative approaches.

The main goals of cancer treatment include:

- Eradication of the cancer

- Control of cancer progression

- Relief of symptoms (palliative care)

- Improvement of quality of life

While some treatments focus on curing the disease, others aim to shrink tumors, manage pain, and extend life. Your specific treatment path will depend on :

- The type and stage of cancer

- Your age and overall health

- Your personal preferences

- Your philosophy toward healing and wellness

Conventional treatments—such as surgery, chemotherapy, radiation, hormone therapy, immunotherapy, and targeted therapies—can be powerful tools, but they also come with risks and side effects, including long-term cellular damage. In some cases, they may even act as carcinogenic agents themselves, increasing the risk of future disease. This makes it all the more important to carefully evaluate the full picture.

Types of conventional treatments

1. Primary treatment: The aim here is to eliminate cancer from the body completely. This is the main treatment strategy—whether through surgery, radiation, or chemotherapy—depending on the cancer type.

2. Adjuvant therapy: This approach follows the primary treatment and seeks to destroy any remaining cancer cells that could cause recurrence. This includes radiation, chemotherapy, or hormone therapy used post-surgery.

3. Neo-adjuvant therapy: Administered before the primary treatment to shrink tumors and make the main therapy (usually surgery) more effective.

4. Palliative treatment: Palliative care doesn't aim to cure but to relieve symptoms and side effects, improving the patient's comfort and quality of life. This is often used in advanced cancer stages, but also alongside curative treatments to help manage pain, fatigue, or emotional distress.

What to expect during treatment

Your treatment journey will be uniquely shaped by your specific diagnosis, your body's response, and the kind of support system you create. That's why it's critical to work with medical professionals who:

- Listen carefully to your concerns

- Involve you in all decisions

- Are open to integrative options

- Do not pressure or coerce you through fear

Unfortunately, some doctors may fall into the habit of using fear—particularly the fear of death—to pressure patients into treatments they don't fully understand. This can strip patients of their autonomy and hinder their capacity to engage with their own healing process.

You have a voice. You have choices.

The importance of an empowered healing plan

I always encourage my patients to build a comprehensive healing plan that includes:

- A personalized nutritional strategy

- Exercise and movement adapted to their energy levels

- Supplements to fill nutritional gaps

- Mind-body tools such as meditation, breathwork, and guided hypnosis

- Emotional and spiritual support

- And yes—conventional therapies, if chosen, applied mindfully and respectfully to the patient's overall values

This integrative approach often helps patients feel in control, improves their resilience, and increases the chances of a successful and peaceful outcome.

A note on simplicity and wisdom

Many of the holistic tools I teach—like fasting, breathwork, yoga, or plant-based nutrition—are ancient practices. Because they seem "too simple" to compete with modern pharmacology, some patients dismiss them. But don't underestimate the power of natural wisdom.

Cancer is often the result of decades of imbalance. Restoring health requires not just fighting disease, but rebuilding harmony. Simplicity, consistency, and intention can go a long way.

I believe in the body's extraordinary ability to regenerate, and I've seen the results when patients combine modern science with ancient knowledge.

In summary

- Cancer treatment is not one-size-fits-all. Explore every option, ask questions, and build a team that supports your values.

- Work with professionals who make you feel heard, respected, and involved.

- Understand the goals of each treatment: curative, preventative, or palliative.

- Create a healing strategy that includes mind, body, and spirit—not just medication.

- Stay open. The path to healing is unique, but never linear.

Current cancer treatment options: a comprehensive overview

When facing a cancer diagnosis, it's important to understand that there is no single "right" approach—what matters most is making an informed decision tailored to your unique biology, values, and preferences. Modern Western medicine has developed numerous techniques for diagnosing, treating, and managing cancer. Some are aggressive and curative in intent, while others are palliative, aiming to relieve symptoms and improve quality of life.

Below is a guide to the most commonly used conventional cancer treatments, each with its benefits, risks, and evolving innovations.

1. Radiation therapy

Radiation therapy uses high-energy beams to kill or shrink cancer cells by damaging their DNA. It can be delivered in two main ways:

- External beam radiation therapy: A machine delivers X-rays, gamma rays, or protons from outside the body, targeting a specific area.

- Internal radiation therapy (brachytherapy): Radioactive material is implanted directly inside or near the tumor.

Radiation is often used in combination with surgery or chemotherapy and is highly localized, meaning it affects primarily the targeted tissue—but healthy tissue nearby can also be affected.

2. Clinical trials

Clinical trials are research-based treatment protocols designed to test new therapies, drug combinations, or medical devices. Participating in a clinical trial may give you access to the latest scientific advances, often years before they become widely available. Trials also play a key role in shaping future treatment standards.

Always ask your oncologist about ongoing trials appropriate for your diagnosis and whether you are eligible to participate.

3. Cryoablation

Cryoablation destroys cancer cells through extreme cold. A thin probe (cryoprobe) is inserted into the tumor under imaging guidance. A freezing agent—such as liquid nitrogen or argon gas—is delivered, freezing the cancer tissue. The tissue is then allowed to thaw, and the cycle is repeated, causing cellular rupture and death.

Cryoablation is especially useful for small, localized tumors, and is sometimes used in prostate, liver, and breast cancers.

4. Radiofrequency ablation (RFA)

RFA kills cancer cells by delivering radiofrequency electrical energy via a needle electrode inserted directly into the tumor. The high-frequency current generates heat (around 60–100°C), destroying cancer cells.

It's typically used for small tumors in the liver, lungs, kidneys, or bones, especially when surgery is not possible.

5. Surgery

Surgery remains one of the most effective ways to physically remove cancerous tissue, especially if the tumor is localized. It may be used alone or in conjunction with chemotherapy or radiation.

Types of cancer surgeries include:
- Curative surgery (removal of tumor)

- Debulking surgery (removing as much of the tumor as possible)

- Palliative surgery (relieving symptoms)

- Reconstructive surgery (e.g., after mastectomy)

6. Immunotherapy

Also called biological therapy, immunotherapy works by activating or enhancing your own immune system to recognize and attack cancer cells. This can involve:

- Checkpoint inhibitors

- CAR-T cell therapy

- Cytokine therapy

- Cancer vaccines

While promising, not all patients respond to immunotherapy. It tends to be more effective in cancers like melanoma, lung cancer, and some blood cancers.

7. Hormone therapy

Certain cancers—such as breast, prostate, ovarian, and endometrial cancers—grow in response to hormones. Hormone therapy either:

- Blocks hormone receptors in cancer cells

- Lowers the body's hormone levels

By cutting off this hormonal "fuel," the growth of cancer cells can be slowed or stopped altogether.

8. Chemotherapy

Chemotherapy uses cytotoxic drugs to target rapidly dividing cells, including cancer cells. It can be systemic (affecting the entire body) or localized. However, its drawback is that it often harms healthy cells, especially in the bone marrow, digestive tract, and hair follicles.

There are two general approaches:

- Maximum Tolerated Dose (MTD): A high-dose strategy intended to kill as many cancer cells as possible. While it can be initially effective, it often leaves behind resistant cancer cells that can later return more aggressively.

- Metronomic or Fractionated Chemotherapy: This involves low-dose, frequent administration, aiming to reduce side effects and target cancer cell angiogenesis (formation of blood vessels that feed tumors). Research shows it may be especially effective when combined with other supportive therapies.

9. Targeted drug therapy

This therapy zeroes in on specific genetic mutations or proteins unique to cancer cells. These "smart drugs" interrupt the processes that allow cancer cells to grow, divide, and evade death.

Examples include:

- Tyrosine kinase inhibitors (e.g., Imatinib)

- PARP inhibitors for BRCA-mutated cancers

- Monoclonal antibodies

10. Bone Marrow transplant (stem cell transplant)

Used primarily in blood cancers like leukemia, lymphoma, and multiple myeloma, this treatment involves replacing damaged bone marrow with healthy stem cells—either from the patient (autologous) or a donor (allogeneic).

It allows for high-dose chemotherapy to be administered and can re-establish the body's ability to produce blood cells.

Immune regeneration and the recalibration of the tumor ecosystem

For much of modern oncology, cancer has been approached as an enemy to eliminate. Surgery removes. Chemotherapy destroys. Radiation damages. Targeted therapies block. The dominant metaphor has been war.

Yet an emerging therapeutic framework is shifting that metaphor—from destruction alone to restoration and recalibration.

This approach does not deny the importance of eradication strategies. Instead, it asks a more fundamental question:

What if cancer persists not only because malignant cells grow uncontrollably, but because the immune system has been rendered functionally ineffective within the tumor environment?

Rather than focusing exclusively on killing cancer cells, this model aims to restore immune competence at the cellular level.

Cancer as Immune Suppression

In this emerging view, cancer is not solely a genetic malfunction. It is also a disease of immune evasion.

Tumors do not simply grow—they actively reshape their surroundings. They alter cytokine signaling, recruit suppressive immune cells, exhaust cytotoxic T-cells, and create microenvironments that dampen immune surveillance.

The result is not an absent immune response, but a silenced one.

The regenerative goal, therefore, becomes functional:□ to awaken and recalibrate immune recognition.

Therapeutic immune education:

Central to this framework is the concept of therapeutic immune education.

Unlike preventive vaccines, which prepare the immune system to avoid future infection, therapeutic cancer vaccines attempt to present tumor-specific antigens in a way that reactivates cytotoxic immune pathways.

The process involves:

Identifying tumor-associated or patient-specific antigens

Delivering these antigens through immune-stimulating platforms

Activating dendritic cells

Expanding tumor-reactive T-cell populations

Overcoming suppressive signals within the microenvironment

The aim is not to replace standard treatment, but to enhance immune surveillance alongside it.

In this sense, regeneration refers not to rebuilding tissue, but to restoring immune function.

The tumor microenvironment as target

Cancer behaves less like an isolated mass and more like an ecosystem.

Within that ecosystem:

Myeloid-derived suppressor cells inhibit T-cell activation

Regulatory T-cells blunt immune attack

Inflammatory cytokines distort signalling

Metabolic competition weakens immune cells

If immune cells cannot function within this environment, even highly targeted therapies may have limited durability.

Thus, emerging strategies seek to:

Reduce immune suppression

Improve antigen presentation

Enhance T-cell persistence

Support long-term immune memory

The objective is not temporary tumor shrinkage, but sustained immune competence.

Regeneration as functional restoration

It is important to clarify what regeneration means in this context.

It does not imply regrowth of damaged tissue or replacement of organs.

It refers to the restoration of cellular intelligence—particularly immune recognition and communication.

This represents a subtle but profound shift.

Instead of viewing cancer exclusively as rogue cells to eliminate, this model sees it as a failure of coordinated cellular defence.

Restoring coordination may be as critical as destroying malignancy.

Integration with conventional Oncology

These emerging approaches are not designed as stand-alone cures. They are most often explored in combination with:

Chemotherapy

Radiation

Checkpoint inhibitors

Targeted molecular therapies

When tumors are disrupted by conventional treatment, they may release antigens that become more visible to an activated immune system.

The synergy between disruption and immune recalibration may define the next era of oncology.

Early signals and ongoing questions

Preliminary clinical investigations suggest potential improvements in immune activation markers and, in some cases, durability of response when immune-educating strategies are combined with standard therapies.

However, important questions remain:

Which patients benefit most?

How durable are immune responses?

What biomarkers predict success?

How can immune-related toxicity be minimized?

These approaches remain under active investigation and require continued peer-reviewed validation.

Innovation must remain tethered to evidence.

The emerging paradigm

One prominent figure associated with this immune-regenerative framework is Dr. Patrick Soon-Shiong, whose work has emphasized tumor-immune mapping, antigen presentation, and personalized immune activation. His efforts represent part of a broader shift toward systems-level oncology.

The larger implication extends beyond any one researcher.

Cancer may increasingly be understood not only as genetic mutation, but as immune miscommunication.

If that hypothesis proves durable, the future of oncology may include:

Personalized immune education

Adaptive vaccine platforms

Microenvironment modulation

AI-driven tumor-immune interaction mapping

The future may not belong solely to eradication strategies, but to intelligent recalibration of biological systems.

In that vision, regeneration does not compete with destruction—it complements it.

It restores what cancer has silenced.

My favorite complementary and natural therapies

Now that we've explored the medical landscape, let's revisit the powerful natural therapies that can support or even amplify your healing journey.

Diet

Nutrition is foundational to cancer prevention and healing. A balanced, plant-forward diet helps maintain a healthy weight, supports immune function, and reduces inflammation.

Research shows that obesity significantly increases the risk of various cancers, including:

- Breast (post-menopausal)

- Endometrial

- Esophageal

- Pancreatic

- Colorectal

- Kidney

Mechanisms include:

- Increased levels of insulin and IGF-1 (growth factors)

- Elevated estrogen from fat tissue

- Chronic low-grade inflammation

Start with a gentle detox to eliminate processed foods, sugars, and alcohol-Focus on whole foods, anti-inflammatory fats, cruciferous vegetables, and fiber-Consider intermittent fasting or a 12:12 eating window to regulate glucose and support autophagy

Supplements, meditation & the Hypnocell® method: enhancing recovery through integrative approaches

In the journey through cancer diagnosis, treatment, and recovery, many patients seek additional tools that go beyond conventional medicine. Among the most promising are targeted supplements, mind-body practices, and subconscious healing techniques. This chapter focuses on how these integrative therapies—when used wisely—can support physical health, ease emotional distress, and possibly enhance overall outcomes.

Supplements: powerful allies when used wisely

There is growing clinical evidence that certain nutritional supplements can:

- Lower the risk of cancer recurrence

- Reduce the side effects of chemotherapy, radiation, or immunotherapy

- Improve energy, immune function, and healing outcomes

- Enhance quality of life in patients during and after treatment

A 2022 review in Frontiers in Pharmacology reported that select vitamins, minerals, and botanicals demonstrated anti-inflammatory, antioxidant, and immunomodulatory properties that support standard cancer care.

Important note: Always consult your oncologist, integrative physician, or clinical nutritionist before introducing supplements—some may interfere with medications or therapies.

Key Supplements worth discussing with your medical team:

1. Vitamin D3

- Low vitamin D levels have been associated with increased cancer risk, especially in colorectal, breast, and prostate cancers.

- Recommended serum levels: 40–60 ng/mL

- Dosage: 1,000–5,000 IU/day (adjusted per blood work)

2. Omega-3 Fatty Acids (EPA/DHA)

- Anti-inflammatory, support cardiovascular and cognitive health

- Can help counteract cachexia (weight loss) and inflammation in cancer patients

3. Curcumin (Turmeric Extract)

- Natural anti-inflammatory and antioxidant

- Shown to sensitize tumor cells to chemotherapy and radiation

4. Mushroom Extracts (Reishi, Turkey Tail, Shiitake)

- Contain beta-glucans that stimulate immune function

- Turkey Tail (PSK) is approved in Japan as an adjunct to cancer therapy

5. Probiotics & Digestive Enzymes

- Essential for gut health, especially after antibiotic use or chemotherapy

- A balanced microbiome improves immune modulation and nutrient absorption

6. Melatonin

- More than a sleep aid—has anti-cancer properties, especially in hormone-related cancers

- May reduce toxicity from radiation and chemotherapy

7. Coenzyme Q10 (CoQ10)

- Supports cellular energy (mitochondria), especially in cardiac tissue

- Can be helpful in fatigue and chemotherapy-related heart complications

8. Glutamine

- May help with mucositis, neuropathy, and GI issues caused by chemotherapy or radiation

9. Magnesium

- Critical for over 300 cellular processes

- Helps reduce muscle cramps, fatigue, and stress response

Supplements to use with caution or avoid:

- High-dose antioxidants (e.g., Vitamin C, E) during radiation or chemotherapy, unless supervised—these may interfere with oxidative stress mechanisms required to kill cancer cells.

- Iron supplements, unless deficient—iron feeds both healthy cells and cancer cells.

For personalized supplement protocols, integrative oncology clinics often offer nutritional genomics testing to tailor recommendations based on your biology.

Meditation & mindfulness: rewiring the mind, rebuilding the Body

When facing cancer, the mind can either become a source of fear and overwhelm, or a powerful partner in healing.

Stress, trauma, and emotional suppression are known to weaken immune function, dysregulate cortisol, and increase systemic inflammation—all of which interfere with recovery.

Benefits of daily meditation practice for cancer patients:

- Reduces anxiety, depression, and cortisol levels

- Improves sleep, pain management, and fatigue

- Enhances focus, optimism, and emotional resilience

- Strengthens immune activity (e.g., natural killer cells)

Evidence: The Mindfulness-Based Stress Reduction (MBSR) protocol has been studied in cancer patients across many trials. A 2021 meta-analysis published in Psycho-Oncology showed significant reductions in stress and improvements in quality of life among patients practicing daily mindfulness.

Start with 5–10 minutes daily, using breath awareness, body scan, or loving-kindness techniques. Apps like Insight Timer, Calm, or Headspace are excellent starting points.

The power of the subconscious mind: Hypnocell® & cellular regeneration

Only about 10% of our thoughts are conscious. The remaining 90% live in the subconscious, storing our beliefs, memories, fears, and automatic responses. If your subconscious is holding on to fear, trauma, or resignation, your body may unconsciously resist healing.

This is where my program, Hypnocell®, comes in.

I developed Hypnocell® as a fusion of:
- Clinical hypnosis

- Cellular biology

- Trauma-informed healing

- Meditative neuro-reprogramming

Hypnocell® helps access deep layers of the subconscious and reprogram internal messages that may be sabotaging recovery. This method has been used successfully with patients facing:
- Cancer

- Autoimmune disorders

- Emotional trauma

- Chronic inflammation and pain

How Hypnocell® works:

1. Guided hypnotic induction to bypass conscious resistance

2. Targeted affirmations and imagery related to cellular regeneration, immune strength, and DNA healing

3. Emotional release and trauma reprocessing, freeing stuck biological patterns

4. Post-hypnotic suggestions to reinforce positive behaviors and reduce treatment side effects

No adverse side effects. Patients often report deep relaxation, improved sleep, reduced pain, and emotional clarity after just a few sessions.

You can explore the full program and testimonials at:

Final note before moving forward

Whether you're newly diagnosed or in recovery, combining medical treatments with natural and mind-body therapies gives you the most robust foundation for healing.

Always keep your team informed. Build your inner circle with professionals who respect your values, and allow yourself to become a full participant in your healing—not just a recipient of treatment.

In the next chapter, we'll explore how to build your support system, ask for help, and create boundaries that protect your energy during this transformative time.

Chapter 7
Cellular Regeneration

Perhaps it's my lifelong refusal to accept life in black and white, my persistent pursuit of the light at the end of every tunnel, that led me to the profound discovery of cellular regeneration.

I've always been one of those people who, upon hearing "You can't do that," "It's not possible," or "There's no evidence for that," feel only more inspired to look deeper. That rebellious spark—fueled by empathy and curiosity—is what eventually allowed me to connect the seemingly invisible threads between the mind, the body, and the cells that make us who we are.

A personal journey through mind and medicine

When I began my deeper journey into the mysteries of the human mind, I was still operating mostly from my left, logical brain. As a doctor and a scientist, I was trained to seek measurable, peer-reviewed, observable evidence. But what I saw, what I experienced—both in patients and in myself—went far beyond what textbooks could explain.

I sought out the best mentors and guides I could find, those who had crossed the threshold into fields that blended psychology, biology, quantum physics, and ancient wisdom. From them, I learned to see the mind as a multidimensional operating system, with hidden control panels that most of us never even access.

That's when everything began to change.

The three levels of the mind

To understand cellular regeneration, we must first understand how the mind interfaces with the body.

1. The conscious mind

This is the part most of us are familiar with—the rational, decision-making mind. It governs what we are aware of at any given moment: what to wear, what to eat, what to say, which show to watch. But this part of the mind only accounts for about 10% of our cognitive power.

2. The subconscious mind

This is the bridge between the conscious and the unconscious. It stores memories, automatic responses, belief systems, and deeply embedded emotional patterns. It is also the master regulator of our physiology—breathing, digestion, cell repair, immune response—all of which happen without our conscious input.

But here's the key: your subconscious doesn't forget anything. Especially not the emotionally charged experiences of your early life.

3. The unconscious mind

This is the deep well of instincts, inherited programming, trauma, and cellular memory—where disease, healing, identity, and ancestral patterns reside.

The subconscious and unconscious mind are the hidden architects of our health. And unless we consciously engage with them, they will continue to run our lives—and our biology—on autopilot.

The early years: programming health or disease

Up until the age of 7, a child's brain operates mostly in theta brainwave state—a deeply absorbent, hypnotic state. Children don't filter information like adults; they feel, absorb, and record emotional patterns based on the environment around them.

At this stage:

- Every word, tone, touch, and absence of affection is encoded.

- Positive responses are integrated as confidence and emotional resilience.

- Negative responses—neglect, rejection, fear, shame—are stored and locked away in the subconscious as a form of protection.

These early emotional roots form the foundation of one's adult health. When unresolved, they can express themselves decades later as chronic illness, autoimmunity, or in some cases, cancer.

"The body keeps the score." – Dr. Bessel van der Kolk

The roots of disease begin long before diagnosis

Cancer is not a sudden event. It's the culmination of years, often decades, of cellular dysregulation. While lifestyle, toxins, genetics, and environmental factors all play roles, so too do suppressed emotions, subconscious beliefs, and unresolved trauma.

Modern epigenetics now confirms what holistic healers have long intuited: environment and experience can turn genes on or off.

The first disease officially linked to epigenetic changes was cancer in 1983. Since then, thousands of studies have shown that trauma, stress, beliefs, and emotions alter gene expression, protein synthesis, and immune modulation.

The body remembers

Cells have memory.

Not just the memory of physical injuries, but of emotional wounds, psychological imprints, and energetic experiences. These memories, stored in the subconscious and in the quantum field of the body, can either foster regeneration or feed degeneration.

That's where cellular regeneration becomes a radical—and essential—approach to healing.

What is cellular regeneration?

Cellular regeneration is the natural process by which the body repairs, restores, and replaces damaged or aging cells with new, healthy ones. It is how we heal a cut, recover from the flu, and rebuild tissues after injury.

But this process can be accelerated, inhibited, or misdirected depending on:

- Emotional stress and mental patterns

- Nutrition and inflammation

- Environmental toxins

- Hormonal imbalances

- Energetic blockages

In cancer, the regeneration process is often hijacked, leading to uncontrolled cell growth. By accessing the subconscious drivers behind cellular dysfunction, we can reverse the direction, triggering cellular death in malignant cells and regeneration in healthy tissue.

The role of Hypnocell® in cellular healing

My program, Hypnocell®, was born from this realization.

Through hypnosis, guided subconscious reprogramming, **and** cellular visualization, Hypnocell® helps patients:

- Release trauma stored in the body

- Reprogram subconscious beliefs that interfere with healing

- Activate genetic potential for regeneration

- Reconnect with the body's innate intelligence

Hypnocell® is not a replacement for medical treatment, but rather a powerful adjunctive approach that gives patients agency, empowerment, and emotional relief during the healing journey.

You can learn more at .

We are designed to heal

You are not broken.

Your cells are listening.Your subconscious is waiting.Your body is still capable of healing—no matter how long it has been sick.

Cellular regeneration is not a fantasy—it is a biological reality that you can learn to activate, support, and trust.

The influence of generational trauma and childhood experiences on health

Good and peaceful experiences create beautiful memories. People who grow up in emotionally secure environments tend to develop a stronger sense of self-worth, resilience, and optimism. Their inner world becomes a safe place, allowing them to face life's challenges with a sense of agency and purpose. These individuals often go on to live fulfilled and accomplished lives—not necessarily because their lives were easier, but because their early emotional foundations were stronger.

On the other hand, children who were neglected, harshly criticized, blamed, or exposed to toxic dynamics of shame and guilt often carry invisible wounds into adulthood. These wounds may not be visible on the outside, but they leave lasting impressions on a child's subconscious. Over time, these emotional imprints can lead to depressive tendencies, chronic anxiety, or even physical illness.

Many of these suppressed experiences surface during adolescence—a time of emotional volatility when the brain is still developing and the body begins to express unresolved stress from earlier childhood. This stage often marks the first peak of psychosomatic expression, where emotional trauma manifests as chronic symptoms or behavioral disorders.

The role of generational patterns in emotional health

Depending on the generation a person belongs to, they may share emotional imprints, cultural trauma, or behavioral patterns shaped by the collective circumstances of their era. After working with hundreds of patients across various backgrounds and ages, I noticed clear trends: each generation has predominant emotional wounds—and corresponding health issues.

The baby boomers (1946–1964)

This generation was born into a post-war world, still marked by scarcity, rigidity, and strict social norms. While new ideas were beginning to emerge, expression was still heavily suppressed. Discipline, obedience, and conformity were expected. Children who were "different" were often shamed or punished.

During this time, human rights were poorly respected, and children were rarely treated with emotional sensitivity. Many were raised by emotionally unavailable or authoritarian parents. As a result, children in this generation often developed:

- Chronic viral or respiratory infections

- Gastrointestinal disorders

- Neurological sensitivities

- A tendency to suppress emotions, leading to autoimmune diseases or silent chronic illness in later life

This generation learned to "push through," often ignoring their emotional needs—a coping strategy that the body eventually mirrored with illness.

Generation X (1965–1979)

The children of the Baby boomers were born during a period of rapid change—especially technological and social. Gen X witnessed the first waves of digital transformation, economic shifts, and dual-working-parent households. Many experienced emotional neglect, not necessarily out of malice, but due to parents being absent or overburdened.

This generation learned to be independent early, but without the emotional tools to process abandonment or isolation. The result? A rise in emotional fragmentation and identity confusion.

Common issues include:

- Obsessive-compulsive tendencies

- Low self-esteem and chronic guilt

- Suicidal ideation or emotional numbness

- Dependency issues masked as hyper-independence

- A surge in undiagnosed chronic conditions, later managed through quick pharmaceutical fixes

This was the generation where medicine began masking root causes with medications—suppressing symptoms without healing the source.

Millennials (1980–1996)

Millennials were raised in a period that valued emotional awareness more than ever before—but often overcorrected by offering too much protection and comfort. Their parents, many of whom came from hardship, wanted their children to feel loved, safe, and fulfilled. However, without boundaries or resilience-building, many Millennials grew up with unrealistic expectations of happiness.

They were often taught that success and comfort were external: found in career, material things, or praise. But when these external markers didn't provide true satisfaction, many were left feeling disillusioned, empty, or deeply anxious.

Emotional patterns often seen in this generation:

- High rates of anxiety, depression, and existential crises

- A persistent sense of "not enoughness"

- Spiritual detachment and emotional dysregulation

- Increasing rates of autoimmune disorders, migraines, chronic fatigue, and even early metabolic issues

Their suffering is internal and subtle—deep, but often hidden behind curated social media lives and high-functioning anxiety.

The lasting imprint of childhood

As you can see, every generation carries its own trauma, shaped by collective events, parenting styles, and cultural pressures. Unfortunately, children absorb the brunt of these energies, and their first 7 years are the most critical period in shaping future physical and emotional health.

During early childhood:

- The brain is operating mostly in theta state (a deeply suggestible, emotional state)

- Children record everything as truth, even if it's not logical

- Experiences of rejection, fear, abandonment, or shame are stored as "core beliefs" that shape adult behaviors—and health

These stored beliefs form the framework of the subconscious mind, which governs 90–95% of our actions, behaviors, and physiological responses.

The deep waters of the subconscious

Not all memories are accessible. Some are readily retrievable (e.g., a birthday, a favorite teacher, a familiar smell), while others are locked away in the deep subconscious—buried for survival. This is a coping mechanism, meant to protect us from emotional overload. But the emotional residue remains and can emerge later in life as illness or self-sabotage.

The deeper the trauma, the more hidden it becomes, often requiring professional methods like hypnosis, EMDR, or somatic therapy to bring it to the surface.

The unconscious mind: the gateway to the higher self

Beyond the subconscious lies the unconscious mind—a realm of archetypes, ancestral memory, primitive emotion, and spiritual insight. This level is often inaccessible through logic alone. Some call this the seat of the soul or the channel to the higher self.

In hypnotherapy, this is where the most profound transformation takes place. When we tap into this space, we access the root of our illness, our hidden beliefs about life, and even our deepest capacity for healing.

Healing is possible

By understanding your generational blueprint and how your early emotional experiences shaped your health, you can begin the process of rewriting your story—at the cellular level.

You are not doomed by your childhood.You are not limited by your parents' pain.And you are not bound by the traumas of your generation.

With intention, awareness, and the right tools, you can heal—deeply, and fully.

Accessing the deeper levels of the mind: the key to cellular regeneration

So how do we access these profound levels of the mind?

That was the central question that launched my deepest research journey. Once I realized the enormous influence the subconscious and unconscious mind have over the physical body, I knew I had to find a way to safely and effectively reach those layers—because that's where true healing begins.

I had already seen how emotions, especially unprocessed ones from childhood, could anchor themselves into the cellular structure of the body. These emotional memories are not just "in the head"—they're encoded in our biology. When the mind locks away trauma, guilt, shame, or fear, the cells store the residue, creating energetic imprints that can manifest as chronic illness over time.

As I dove into this work, I learned that some emotional roots are shallow—they can be uncovered and processed quickly. But others run very deep, tangled around one's earliest years and shaped by generational trauma, emotional neglect, or significant life events. Accessing and rewiring these deep-rooted experiences requires knowledge, patience, and a profound understanding of both psychology and cellular behavior.

From embryology to emotional healing

Working for years as an embryologist gave me a unique lens. I've spent countless hours observing the behavior and development of cells at their earliest stages—cells that are pure, undifferentiated, and unburdened by trauma. And it's fascinating: embryonic cells, though young, are often more complex in their behavior than adult cells. They're in constant communication, orchestrating a dance of growth and specialization.

This early work with embryos laid the foundation for my understanding of how trauma alters communication between cells later in life. By the time someone is facing a chronic illness—or a cancer diagnosis—those communication pathways have often been disrupted by years of unresolved emotional imprinting.

So how do we reach these levels of the mind?

The mind is not one singular structure. It is composed of layers, each with its own language and access point:

- The conscious mind handles logic, choice, and awareness.

- The subconscious mind stores memories, emotional reactions, patterns, and belief systems—especially those formed before the age of seven.

- The unconscious mind is the deepest layer, housing ancestral memory, primal instincts, and the connection to your higher self.

To truly access the subconscious and unconscious levels, we must go beyond logic and language. There are two main techniques I have found highly effective:

1. Meditation

Meditation, especially when practiced daily, helps calm the nervous system and gently lower the brainwave frequency from beta (active thought) to alpha and theta states—where subconscious programming resides.

A regular practice of 5 to 10 minutes a day can:

- Lower stress hormones like cortisol

- Balance immune response

- Improve sleep and healing outcomes

- Begin unlocking surface-level subconscious content

Meditation creates the conditions for the mind and body to return to balance. It's accessible, free, and scientifically backed.

2. Hypnosis and the Hypnocell® Method

For deeper work—where we need to uncover and reprogram deeply rooted emotional patterns—I developed Hypnocell®, a method that combines clinical hypnosis with insights from cell biology, neuroplasticity, and trauma healing.

This method has been transformative. It guides patients into the subconscious mind, where they can safely recall, reframe, and release experiences that have been silently shaping their biology for decades.

In some cases, the process may take a few sessions. In more deeply embedded cases, it can take up to six months of regular work. But once the message is implanted and accepted by the subconscious, the healing cascade begins. Cells begin to regenerate. Inflammation reduces. Symptoms fade. It's a beautiful, tangible transformation.

But what about terminal patients?

Many people ask: "What about patients who have been told they only have weeks to live?"

I have worked with terminally ill patients—those given little hope by the medical system—and what I've seen is remarkable.

We begin by integrating detoxification, plant-based nutrition, supplementation, exercise, and meditation at their own pace. At the same time, we engage in Hypnocell® sessions to address emotional roots and plant new regenerative instructions into the subconscious mind.

The result?

- Improved symptom control

- Greater emotional peace and acceptance

- In some cases, partial remission or full remission

While I cannot promise that 100% of patients will fully recover, I can say with confidence that a significant percentage show clinical improvement—and, most importantly, they experience a restored sense of power and peace.

The mind: the foundation of healing

I've come to believe, without a doubt, that the mind is a foundational pillar of health—just as important as diet, medication, or surgery. You can have the best treatment plan in the world, but if your subconscious mind believes you're broken, guilty, or hopeless... the body will respond accordingly.

Conversely, when you empower the subconscious with healing beliefs, the immune system becomes more efficient, inflammation decreases, and the body begins to heal.

Next steps

If you're a patient—or someone supporting a patient—who is ready to begin this work, you can explore:

- My courses and resources at

- Hypnocell® programs and information at

- Free meditations and support tools designed specifically for patients

A final thought

I have found that every single patient I've treated using Hypnocell® has shown a memory, belief, or experience rooted in their early years—most often before the age of seven. That period, when the subconscious is most active, sets the tone for a person's emotional and physical life.

Your story didn't start with your diagnosis.

But it can change now.

With the right tools, awareness, and support, you can access the deepest levels of your mind, and begin to truly heal—cell by cell, thought by thought.

Chapter 8
Always seek help

From the very beginning of this book, I've emphasized one powerful truth: no one should face cancer alone.

Whether you're a patient, a loved one, or simply someone wanting to offer support, knowing how to seek help—or how to give it—can make all the difference in the healing process. Science has shown that a strong support system can improve quality of life, increase survival rates, and reduce stress and anxiety in cancer patients. Yet the act of reaching out for help can still feel overwhelming.

In this chapter, we will explore how to seek the right help—and how to be the right help for someone going through the cancer journey.

We'll divide this chapter into two essential sections:

1. For Patients – Empowering actions to seek and receive meaningful support

2. For Friends and Family – Ways to become a truly supportive presence

Part I: If you're a patient – how to ask for and receive help

Receiving a cancer diagnosis can feel like the ground has shifted beneath your feet. There are emotional waves of fear, grief, confusion, and sometimes anger. But amid the storm, there is always the possibility of healing, peace, and strength—especially when you're not alone.

Let's explore some ways you can take ownership of your healing journey while surrounding yourself with the right kind of support:

1. Join a support group

One of the most effective and healing actions you can take is to connect with others who truly understand what you're going through.

Support groups are not about complaining—they are about community, courage, and shared wisdom. They provide a space where fears can be spoken without judgment, and where hope is passed from one patient to another.

Look for groups at local hospitals, wellness centers, or even online. Many cancer centers now offer both in-person and virtual support circles, sometimes organized by cancer type, age, or treatment stage. Some are led by therapists or oncology social workers, while others are peer-led.

The greatest gift of joining a support group? Realizing that you are not alone, and never were.

2. Express your feelings—even the hard ones

Many patients find themselves trying to "stay strong" for their loved ones, hiding their pain or fear to avoid burdening others. But bottling up emotions can increase stress, lower immunity, and delay healing.

It's time to give yourself permission to feel—and to share those feelings.

Speak with a friend. Write in a journal. Talk to a therapist or counselor. Join a creative expression group. Vulnerability is not weakness—it's a doorway to healing.

And remember: people can't help you if they don't know what you need. If you're craving a hug, say it. If you're feeling scared, say it. You deserve to be heard, seen, and held—emotionally and physically.

3. Cultivate a positive mindset—even in darkness

Yes, the word "cancer" and the word "positivity" seem incompatible. And no, we're not talking about toxic positivity or pretending everything is okay when it's not. This is about consciously choosing to focus on what's still good, even if it's small.

Did you laugh today? That matters. Did someone make you feel cared for? That counts. Did you get out of bed and try your best? That's courage.

Even the darkest storms give way to rainbows—and sometimes, your new perspective becomes the most powerful part of your healing.

Research has shown that optimism and gratitude can improve immune function, reduce treatment side effects, and enhance emotional resilience. It's not about denying pain—it's about finding meaning and hope through it.

Part II: If you're a loved one – how to truly help

If someone you care about is facing cancer, it's natural to feel helpless at times. You may not know what to say, or you may fear doing or saying the wrong thing. That's okay. Your presence and your willingness to learn already mean more than you think.

Here are some ways you can truly show up:

1. Ask before you act

Instead of jumping in to offer advice or fix things, start by asking:

"What do you need most today?" "How can I support you right now?" "Would you like company, or quiet time?"

Let the patient lead. Empower them with choice.

2. Be consistent and present

People often rally in the beginning, then disappear as the journey continues. But cancer doesn't go away after the first round of treatment. Long-term support matters.

Send a text just to say you're thinking of them. Drop off a favorite tea. Offer a ride to a treatment session—or just sit quietly and hold their hand.

You don't have to have perfect words. Just show up. Stay steady. Be real.

3. Respect their choices

Some patients choose aggressive treatments. Others pursue integrative or alternative care. Some fight with everything they have; others choose peace and comfort. Your role is not to direct their path, but to support the one they choose.

Be curious, not judgmental. Offer compassion, not correction.

4. Take care of yourself too

Being a caregiver or emotional support can be deeply rewarding—but also draining. You can only give from a full cup.

Make sure you have your own support system. Talk to others who've been through this. Practice self-care. Cry when you need to. You are not expected to carry it all.

Together, we heal

The cancer journey is not just about survival—it's about transformation, resilience, and connection. Patients heal best when they are surrounded by love and empowered by choice. And supporters become stronger, wiser, and more compassionate in the process.

After reading this chapter, I hope you feel more equipped—whether you are the one facing cancer, or walking beside someone who is. We are stronger together. We are wiser when we listen. And we are more powerful than we think—when we ask for help and when we offer it with heart.

4. Spend time with the people you love

Healing doesn't only happen through medicine—it happens through connection. One of the most powerful healing agents is love. Surrounding yourself with people who genuinely care for you, who know your heart and your story, is essential during this time.

Now is not the time to isolate yourself or surround yourself with well-meaning strangers who don't understand the depth of your emotions. Instead, lean into the embrace of those who love you without needing explanations—friends, family, your chosen tribe.

These are the people who will sit with you in silence when words fail, who will make you laugh on your darkest days, and who will help you remember who you are beyond the diagnosis. Be intentional about spending time with them. Let them love you. Let yourself be seen.

5. Be grateful for life—and stop blaming yourself

It's easy to fall into a spiral of "Why me?" when facing a life-altering illness. Many patients experience guilt, self-blame, or even shame. These emotions are completely human—but they are also toxic to healing.

You are not to blame.

Cancer is not a punishment. It is not a failure of will, of diet, of choices. It is a complex, multifactorial condition that can affect anyone.

Practicing gratitude may feel unnatural in the face of illness, but research shows that cultivating gratitude boosts immune function, improves mental health, and increases life satisfaction—even in cancer patients.

Be thankful for the breath in your lungs. For the sunrise. For the kindness of a nurse. For the friend who sent you a funny message. And most of all, be grateful for the opportunity this journey gives you—to awaken, to grow, to live more consciously.

Healing begins when self-blame ends, and love for life returns.

How to support someone with cancer

Being a support system for someone battling cancer is a sacred and powerful role. It's not about having all the answers—it's about being present, compassionate, and consistent.

Here are five ways to support a loved one with cancer:

1. Be emotionally available

Emotional presence means being more than just physically there. It means showing up with empathy and open-heartedness. Let the person express their emotions freely—tears, anger, fear, confusion—and don't rush to "fix" them.

If they cry, hold them.If they're scared, listen without judgment.If they feel lost, remind them that they are still deeply loved.

Being emotionally available often means sitting in silence together, offering comfort simply by being there. Your calm, steady presence is one of the most powerful gifts you can give.

2. Offer rides to appointments (and more)

Hospital appointments can be daunting. Even the most independent person may feel anxious or drained before scans, bloodwork, or treatments. Offering to drive them, accompany them, or simply wait nearby can relieve a massive burden.

This isn't just about logistics—it's about partnership. Your presence gives emotional courage, and helps the patient feel they are not alone on this road.

When I was diagnosed with a brain cavernoma, I initially thought I had to be strong and face all my medical appointments alone. But when friends and family insisted on accompanying me, I felt a wave of calm and reassurance. I didn't realize how much I needed their presence until I experienced the warmth it brought.

We don't always need strength—we need support.

3. Stay consistently connected

Support isn't just for the diagnosis phase—it's needed throughout the entire journey.

It's common for friends to check in during the initial diagnosis and then disappear as time goes on. But healing doesn't happen overnight. Continued support over the weeks and months makes a profound difference.

Text them regularly. Call just to chat. Send a card. Drop off their favorite meal. Invite them to watch a movie together—even if it's virtual. These small actions add up to a feeling of deep, abiding connection.

Your consistent presence says: You matter. I'm still here. You're not forgotten.

4. Avoid over-compensating or over-helping

It's natural to want to "do everything" for someone who's sick—but be mindful of allowing them to retain independence and dignity. Too much assistance can unintentionally reinforce a sense of helplessness.

Instead, strike a balance:

- Help prepare meals, but invite them to join in if they can.

- Offer to clean up, but let them choose what stays and goes.

- Encourage them to walk, cook, or socialize when they feel up to it.

Treat them as capable individuals, not fragile patients. Empower them gently.

5. Motivate, love, and care for them with heart

Above all else, lead with love.

Love is medicine. It transcends fear, softens pain, and creates an atmosphere of safety and hope. Your love doesn't need to be perfect—it just needs to be real.

Encourage them, remind them of their strength, reflect back the light you see in them when they feel lost in the dark. Anticipate their needs, respect their boundaries, and offer your energy without expectation.

And don't forget to manage your own energy. You can't pour from an empty cup. Take care of yourself so that your love remains full, vibrant, and healing.

Love transmits energy. And loving presence can be one of the most potent healing forces in the world.

Final thoughts

Whether you're facing cancer yourself or supporting someone you care about, remember: healing is a collective experience.

Cancer doesn't just test the body—it tests our relationships, our strength, our ability to ask for help, and to give it unconditionally. But within those challenges lies an invitation to deepen connection, compassion, and humanity.

Let us rise to the occasion—with grace, with courage, and with the unshakable belief that none of us are meant to walk this road alone.

Support is not just helpful in the journey through cancer—it is essential. Healing is never one-dimensional. It encompasses physical, emotional, psychological, and even spiritual aspects of the human experience. No one should have to walk this path alone.

In this chapter, we've explored how both cancer patients and their loved ones can take intentional steps to give and receive meaningful support. Whether you're the one facing the diagnosis or the friend standing beside them, your role matters deeply.

If you know someone battling cancer, don't wait for them to ask for help. Sometimes, the strongest people are the least likely to reach out. Take the initiative—show up, offer comfort, stay connected. Your presence can be the lifeline they didn't know they needed.

And if you're a cancer patient, remember: you don't have to do it all alone. Asking for help is not a weakness—it is a powerful act of strength and self-respect.

Be proactive in seeking support, because your healing journey is not meant to be carried in silence or solitude.

As we approach the final chapter of this book, we will reflect on the transformative lessons that come from facing cancer—a journey that, while profoundly challenging, can also bring insight, clarity, growth, and unexpected grace. The next chapter is a tribute to the strength within you and the wisdom you gain from walking through the fire.

Chapter 9
Be your own judge

Life doesn't always unfold as we expect. A cancer diagnosis can feel like a devastating plot twist in the story you were writing—but it can also be a chapter that teaches you the most. This chapter is an invitation to take ownership of your narrative, to hold the pen again, and to become the author and the judge of your healing journey.

Cancer teaches lessons—are you listening?

From the very first moment of diagnosis, a powerful shift begins. Most people are shocked by the strength they discover within themselves when they are forced to confront the unimaginable. Cancer reveals a side of you that perhaps you never met before—a version of yourself that shows up in resilience, grace, and unexpected courage.

- You show up for appointments.

- You take the medications.

- You make lifestyle changes.

- You find ways to keep moving forward.

That's resilience, and it's not something to underestimate. Resilience is not the absence of fear or sadness; it is your ability to rise, adapt, and continue, despite them.

You also begin to notice other things: a deeper appreciation for your medical team, who dedicate their lives to healing others. A renewed awareness of time. A sharpened lens on purpose and values. These are not small things. They are transformations.

Illness can shift perspective—if you let it

Serious illness often triggers deep reflection. You might begin asking yourself difficult but necessary questions:

- Am I living the life I truly want?

- Have I been prioritizing what really matters?

- Did I follow my joy, or just do what I had to do?

- Have I expressed love, or held back?

- What do I want to be remembered for?

These reflections aren't just philosophical. Studies show that patients who engage in meaning-centered therapies experience improved emotional resilience and quality of life during cancer treatment.

So here's the truth: Cancer might interrupt your life—but it also provides a profound invitation to reset.

Choose accountability, not blame

When we say "be your own judge," we're not talking about blame or guilt. This chapter isn't about judging yourself harshly. It's about empowerment through awareness.

- Hold yourself accountable for your intentions, not just your reactions.

- Reflect on how you're responding, not just what you're enduring.

- Ask: How can I grow from this? How can I help someone else?

Yes, you have pain. But within that pain, there may be wisdom, growth, and even a mission. Maybe that mission is to support another person. Maybe it's to share your story. Maybe it's to begin living more fully, not just surviving.

Knowledge is power—and now you have it

This book has given you tools that many people don't have access to—strategies for healing the body, mind, and spirit. You've learned about:

- Cellular regeneration

- Nutrition and detox

- Meditation and Hypnocell®

- Emotional trauma and memory

- Natural therapies that complement Western treatments

- How to build a support system—and be one

So here's the question: Now that you know all this, what will you do with it? "With knowledge comes responsibility."

Become an impact maker

You may be surrounded by others who are just beginning their cancer journey—some more scared or more vulnerable than you. Your presence, your story, and your courage to show up authentically could be the light they need.

Impact doesn't always come through grand gestures. Sometimes it's just showing up, saying, "I've been there. You're not alone."

If you're attending support groups, sharing online, or just meeting others in treatment waiting rooms—start asking the deeper questions:

- "What has cancer taught you so far?"

- "What do you want to change after this?"

- "Who have you become through this process?"

These questions unlock meaning, and meaning transforms pain into purpose.

Five final tips to be your own judge:

1. Define your own metrics of successDon't let test results or medical stats alone define your story. Let your courage, effort, and mindset be your daily victories.

2. Let the pain teach you, not define youYou are not just what happened to you. You are who you choose to become because of it.

3. Surround yourself with empowermentLimit exposure to negativity. Curate your environment with people, practices, and media that uplift and energize you.

4. Make a commitment to help othersPurpose is healing. Even helping one person can reaffirm your strength and humanity.

5. Reclaim your power—every dayYour diagnosis may have changed your plans, but it hasn't taken away your power. Choose every day to live intentionally.

Final words

Being your own judge means deciding what kind of life you want to live now—not "after cancer," not "if I survive," but today. Decide who you want to be, how you want to live, and how you want to love.

This book is not just about surviving cancer—it's about becoming more alive than ever.

And you, dear reader, have everything it takes to thrive.

How to be your own judge and be helpful while dealing with cancer

Dealing with cancer may feel like an all-consuming experience—but it doesn't have to take away your ability to give, connect, or inspire. In fact, the journey can awaken in you a greater sense of meaning, purpose, and strength. This section offers practical, heartfelt ways you can be your own judge—taking ownership of your healing—while also being a source of light for others.

1. Smile and reach out to others

There is power in a smile—especially when it's shared in the middle of adversity. Smiling doesn't mean denying what you're going through; it means choosing to offer warmth to others even when you yourself are in pain.

A smile is a subtle act of resilience. It tells others, "I'm still here. I still believe in connection. And I see you." When you smile at a fellow patient in a waiting room, hospital corridor, or support group, you help create a space where others feel safe enough to open up. That moment of connection may be the light in their darkest day.

Even as you read this now, allow yourself a small smile. Let it serve as a quiet affirmation: "I will be alright."

2. Interact with your doctors and nurses

Healthcare providers—especially those who work with cancer patients—carry a heavy emotional load. While their job is clinical, their hearts are human. They often witness suffering, loss, and triumph all within the same shift.

Take a moment to speak to them as people, not just professionals. Ask about their day. Thank them. Share something positive, even a joke. These small gestures build trust and deepen your connection. More importantly, they create an atmosphere of collaborative healing, where your team becomes a circle of care rather than a hierarchy of instruction.

The medical journey becomes lighter when compassion flows both ways.

3. Volunteer to help someone else

Volunteering while you're still on your own cancer journey might seem counterintuitive—but it can be deeply healing. Studies in psycho-oncology confirm that patients who engage in peer-support roles often experience:

- Improved mental health

- Greater sense of purpose

- Better adherence to treatment

- Reduced feelings of isolation

Volunteering doesn't have to mean physical labor or public speaking. It can be as simple as:

- Calling another patient to check in

- Sharing your story with someone newly diagnosed

- Joining an online support group as a listener

- Helping a peer navigate a hospital visit

What makes your support unique is your shared experience. Unlike others who may only offer sympathy, you offer empathy. You know the terrain. You feel their fears. And that makes your presence powerful.

Many of my own patients who began volunteering during their treatment say it changed everything. They discovered a new identity—not just as "a cancer patient," but as a survivor helping others survive.

4. Revisit and apply the tools from this book

This book wasn't meant to be read once and shelved—it was designed to be a lifelong manual. You might forget parts of it during hard days, and that's okay. Return to the tools. Re-read the chapters. Revisit the breathing techniques, the Hypnocell® method, the suggestions on emotional regulation, nutrition, and spiritual awareness.

Healing is not linear—it's a cycle. The more you revisit and implement these practices, the deeper their impact. Let these pages become your anchor.

Think of it this way: when a pilot learns to fly, they rely on a manual to guide them through turbulence. This book is your flight manual through cancer. Keep it close.

5. Embrace your journey with courage and clarity

To embrace your journey is to stop running from it. It means saying:"Yes, this is happening. And I'm going to face it fully, with eyes wide open."

Some patients try to mentally escape, pretending the diagnosis isn't real or living in the past. While denial can serve as temporary protection, it can also block progress. Real transformation begins the moment you stop asking, "Why me?" and start asking, "What can I learn? How can I grow?"

Embracing your journey means:

- Acknowledging your pain without letting it define you

- Being present with your body, even when it's hurting

- Choosing hope even when the future is uncertain

- Letting go of guilt, regret, and "should-haves"

- Rewriting your story from a place of power

It's like the story of the recovering alcoholic who says, "My healing began the day I accepted my reality." Acceptance is not giving up. It's stepping into the truth so you can work with it—not against it.

Final thoughts: transforming experience into empowerment

From the first chapter to now, this book has taken you through every layer of the cancer journey—physiological, emotional, spiritual, and psychological. If there's one thing I hope you remember, it's this:

Cancer is not the end of your story. It can be the beginning of your greatest transformation.

No two experiences are alike, but every patient has the ability to take control of their response, their growth, and their voice. And for those who love someone with cancer—you, too, hold tremendous power to uplift, stabilize, and walk beside your loved one with compassion and strength.

Let us all rise together—patients, families, friends, and caregivers—and create a new way of facing illness: with community, consciousness, and courage.

You are not just surviving. You are evolving.

Chapter 10

Facing cancer during a pandemic or global health crisis

W hen I was close to completing this book, the world was shaken by the outbreak of COVID-19. As the pandemic unfolded, my inbox filled with messages from patients who were fearful, uncertain, and desperate for answers. Their concerns ranged from how to continue treatment safely to what risks they faced with compromised immune systems. Overnight, the number of telemedicine consultations and virtual support sessions tripled.

This chapter addresses the unique challenges—and opportunities for adaptation—that cancer patients face during times of widespread health emergencies, especially global pandemics. While the coronavirus was the trigger for writing this chapter, the principles shared here can apply to any situation where access to healthcare becomes limited or high-risk, such as during epidemics, natural disasters, or lockdowns.

Why pandemics pose a unique threat to cancer patients

Pandemics present a dual threat to cancer patients:

    1. Increased exposure to infection during hospital visits for chemotherapy, surgery, or routine monitoring.

    2. Decreased access to timely care due to hospital restrictions, staffing

shortages, or supply chain disruptions.

During the early months of COVID-19, hospitals—ironically meant to be places of healing—became high-risk environments. This was especially alarming for immunocompromised individuals, including many undergoing cancer treatment.

Cancer weakens the immune system, and many therapies—such as chemotherapy, radiation, or bone marrow transplants—further reduce the body's natural defenses. For this reason, cancer patients are classified as high-risk during infectious disease outbreaks.

Additionally, respiratory viruses like SARS-CoV-2 (the virus that causes COVID-19) have been shown to cause more severe illness in people with underlying health conditions, particularly those with suppressed or dysregulated immune systems.

Understanding viral exposure and immunity

Coronaviruses are a large family of viruses that can infect both animals and humans. While most strains cause only mild symptoms like the common cold, newer strains (like SARS-CoV-2) can lead to severe respiratory illness, particularly in vulnerable populations.

What made COVID-19 especially dangerous:

- High contagion rate, even from asymptomatic individuals

- Delayed symptoms, making detection difficult

- Aerosol and surface transmission, increasing exposure risks in crowded indoor spaces like hospitals

These factors made it extremely difficult to identify and isolate carriers early. For cancer patients, this meant increased vulnerability in medical settings where they typically feel safest.

Mental health struggles during isolation and uncertainty

Alongside the physical risks, the emotional toll of navigating cancer during a global crisis is profound. The sense of isolation, anxiety about infection, and interruption of treatment can lead to:

- Heightened stress hormones, which negatively impact immune response

- Depression and fear of mortality

- Feelings of helplessness and abandonment

- Post-traumatic stress symptoms during or after recovery

This is why maintaining mental and emotional health during such times becomes just as vital as protecting physical health. Many patients benefit from online therapy, guided meditation, or hypnotherapy sessions (such as those offered in the Hypnocell® program), which can provide emotional grounding and reduce stress hormone overload.

Strategies for cancer patients during a pandemic

1. Leverage telemedicine and virtual care

- Many healthcare systems now offer virtual oncology consults, symptom check-ins, and second opinions.

- Use video platforms to stay in touch with your care team while minimizing hospital visits.

- Ask your doctor if lab tests, prescription refills, and treatment plans can be managed remotely.

2. Prioritize infection prevention

- Follow strict hygiene: frequent handwashing, mask use, and sanitizing surfaces.

- Avoid public spaces and limit contact with visitors.

- Ask caregivers and household members to also practice these measures.

3. Maintain continuity of care

- Never cancel or delay treatment without consulting your oncologist.

- If appointments are postponed, request alternative care options, monitoring tools, or home visits if available.

- Keep a medical folder updated with your latest lab results, diagnosis history, and emergency contacts.

4. Protect mental health

- Engage in regular mindfulness, journaling, or breathing techniques to reduce anxiety.

- Join online support groups to feel less isolated.

- Seek professional guidance if you experience emotional overwhelm, depression, or panic.

The bigger picture: what we learned from COVID-19

COVID-19 revealed weaknesses in global healthcare systems—but also highlighted the resilience and adaptability of patients and caregivers. Cancer patients learned how to advocate for themselves, find new ways to connect with others, and discover strength they didn't know they had.

From a medical standpoint, the pandemic also accelerated:

- The development of remote cancer monitoring technologies (wearables, apps, remote vital tracking)

- Improved infection control protocols for outpatient care

- A wider acceptance of integrative therapies to support immune health and mental wellness

Closing thoughts

No one should have to fight cancer alone—especially during a pandemic. But when isolation, fear, and uncertainty knock at the door, you can face them with knowledge, preparation, and community.

If you are living with cancer during a time of global upheaval, remember:

- You have a right to safe and continuous care.

- You are not alone—virtual communities and support systems are only a click away.

- Your body is not just a battleground; it's a healing space that responds to calm, care, and consistency.

Stay informed, stay connected, and never forget that your story matters—especially now.

Until science brings us more definitive answers, there are thoughtful, proactive steps that patients with chronic conditions—especially cancer—can take to protect themselves while continuing their care.

Recent health reports from across Europe have highlighted that many of the early pandemic-related deaths occurred in long-term care facilities, underscoring the importance of enhanced protection and monitoring for vulnerable individuals.

Additionally, a study from China observed that cancer patients who had recently undergone chemotherapy or surgery appeared to face a higher risk of complications from viral infections compared to those not receiving active treatment. Similarly, data from institutions like UCSF Health confirm that patients currently in treatment are generally at higher risk than those in remission.

However, none of this is a reason to panic—it is a reason to prepare.

Empowering yourself with the right actions

The single most important step you can take is to stay in regular communication with your healthcare provider. If you notice any changes in your health—no matter how minor—reach out to your medical team. They are your partners in care and will guide you on whether to visit the clinic or hospital, or whether it's safe and effective to manage things remotely.

If in-person treatment is needed, your medical provider will give you precise instructions on how to protect yourself, including safety protocols, appointment scheduling, and any special precautions. Hospitals and clinics have implemented comprehensive safety procedures to minimize exposure and ensure that patients receive care in the safest way possible.

Embracing the power of telemedicine

If you are not in immediate need of in-person treatment, telemedicine is an excellent option that allows you to stay connected to your care team from the comfort and safety of your home. This service has become one of the most positive transformations in modern healthcare, offering real-time access to medical consultations, treatment updates, and emotional support—all through your phone or computer.

As a practitioner myself, I've worked with telemedicine for many years and have witnessed firsthand how this method empowers patients, enhances communication, and significantly reduces unnecessary exposure. It is truly the future of healthcare for millions of people, and a valuable tool in your healing journey.

When in doubt, ask

If you're unsure about your treatment schedule, safety precautions, or your current level of risk, always consult your physician. Every patient is unique, and doctors tailor their decisions based on your specific needs, history, and current health status. There's no one-size-fits-all when it comes to your well-being.

Avoid self-diagnosing, delaying necessary care, or ignoring medical advice out of fear. This is a time for cooperation, not isolation. Work together with your care team to make wise, informed decisions that prioritize your healing and protection.

Staying safe without fear

It's natural to feel uncertain during a time when an invisible threat seems to loom around us. But remember, knowledge and preparation are the antidotes to fear.

By following evidence-based precautions, staying in contact with your doctor, and utilizing telemedicine and support networks, you can safely navigate your treatment journey with strength and confidence.

This is not a moment to isolate in fear—it's a moment to rise with awareness, to protect yourself smartly, and to embrace the evolving tools that keep us connected, informed, and empowered.

The invisible doesn't mean harmless

Just because you can't see this virus doesn't mean it isn't there.

For those of you currently navigating the already challenging path of cancer treatment, the added stress of a viral pandemic can feel overwhelming. An invisible enemy—an airborne virus—seeks every possible opportunity to spread. But knowledge, preparation, and action are your most powerful defenses.

If you're living with cancer, I want to share some updated and practical advice to help you stay protected, grounded, and emotionally strong during times like these:

1. Follow strict hygiene measures

Regardless of your diagnosis, you must adopt the general health guidelines advised for all—consistently and without exception:

- Wash your hands thoroughly with soap and water for at least 20 seconds.

- Avoid touching your face, particularly your eyes, nose, and mouth, especially when outside your home.

- Wear a high-quality protective mask (such as N95 or KN95) in public spaces or hospitals.

- Maintain physical distance from people, especially those showing cold, flu, or viral symptoms.

- Disinfect high-touch surfaces regularly, including phones, doorknobs, and counters.

These may sound simple, but they are powerful, science-backed tools in limiting viral transmission.

2. Consult your doctor for personalized guidance

Your healthcare provider is your best ally. Speak with your doctor to understand:

- How your current cancer treatment (chemotherapy, radiation, immunotherapy, etc.) may affect your risk.

- Whether appointments can be shifted to telehealth visits.

- How to safely proceed with in-person treatments if necessary.

- What warning signs to look for in relation to COVID-19 or other infections, given your medical history.

Don't hesitate to ask questions. This is your health, and your peace of mind matters.

3. Immediately report symptoms

If you experience symptoms such as fever, fatigue, shortness of breath, persistent cough, or sudden loss of taste/smell:

- Call your doctor right away—do not delay.

- Clearly mention your cancer diagnosis and any immunosuppressive treatments you're receiving.

- Request priority screening and guidance based on your situation.

Early detection can make a significant difference in outcomes.

4. Join a support network

Don't go through this alone. There are cancer-specific mental health and peer support groups available virtually—many created specifically for patients coping with uncertainty during health crises.

These groups provide:

- Emotional relief

- A chance to share and learn from others

- Tools to manage fear, anxiety, and isolation

Look for certified cancer coaches, teletherapy services, and online wellness communities that align with your needs.

5. Engage in calming activities

Being glued to the news can increase anxiety. Try to give your mind a break:

- Practice mindfulness, meditation, or breathing exercises.

- Reconnect with creative hobbies like journaling, painting, or gardening.

- Explore uplifting audiobooks or music playlists.

- Try gentle movement or yoga for cancer patients (many classes are now available online).

These small, mindful practices can help regulate your nervous system and provide a sense of stability.

6. Boost your immunity with nutrition

While no diet can guarantee protection, a well-balanced, immune-supportive diet can strengthen your body and mood:

- Emphasize fresh vegetables, berries, lean proteins, healthy fats like olive oil, and plenty of water.

- Include zinc, selenium, and vitamin C-rich foods, unless otherwise advised by your physician.

- Consider consulting a nutritionist specialized in oncology for tailored recommendations.

7. Stay informed—but wisely

Look for credible, science-based updates regarding cancer care during pandemics from:

- The American Cancer Society

- National Cancer Institute (NCI)

- World Health Organization (WHO)

- Your hospital's oncology department

Stay informed—but don't overwhelm yourself with media overload.

8. Protect your home environment

If you live with others:

- Avoid close contact, especially if anyone is experiencing symptoms.

- Use separate utensils, linens, and bathroom space if possible.

- Encourage household members to follow strict hygiene and distancing when returning home from outside.

If possible, designate a "safe zone" in your home where you can feel relaxed and protected.

9. Coordinate medication deliveries

Reach out to your local pharmacy to arrange home delivery of your prescriptions. Many now offer contactless services and automatic refills, reducing your need to leave home.

Final thoughts

We are living through an extraordinary chapter in human history. Healthcare systems are working tirelessly to manage the needs of vulnerable populations—and that includes you.

Remember:

- Common sense is powerful.

- Protective routines are empowering.

- Staying connected to your care team is vital.

Telemedicine and remote monitoring are not temporary fixes—they're part of a new era in compassionate, accessible care. While we wait for a new normal to emerge, let's continue to adapt wisely and live fully.

A collective awakening

The global pandemic has shown us how interconnected we are, and how fragile yet resilient life can be. When this passes—and it will—we will step into a world more attuned to the importance of prevention, public health, and emotional well-being.

Your journey matters. Your story matters.

Let's face tomorrow not with fear, but with hope, intention, and courage.

Conclusion

A new beginning

You've just completed an important journey—one that has taken you through the depths of understanding cancer not just as a disease, but as a life-altering experience that demands awareness, resilience, and action.

Whether you are a patient, a caregiver, a healthcare professional, or simply someone wanting to be better informed—you have now equipped yourself with valuable knowledge that has the potential to change lives, starting with your own.

But while this may be the final chapter of the book, it is by no means the end of your journey. In fact, this is where your transformation truly begins.

What happens now?

It's easy to close a book and move on to the next thing. But when it comes to health—especially cancer—passive knowledge isn't enough. You must engage. Reflect. Act.

Ask yourself:

- What will I do differently starting today?

- How can I support myself or others more intentionally?

- Which parts of this book resonated the most—and how will I apply them?

This isn't just about absorbing facts. This is about owning your health, your story, and your potential to shape a better outcome.

Knowledge + Action = Transformation

Throughout these chapters, you've learned how cancer begins, how to reduce your risks, what to do if you or someone you love is diagnosed, and how to build a powerful support network.

You've also explored mental, emotional, and cellular approaches to healing—such as meditation, nutrition, self-awareness, and my Hypnocell® method.

But none of this matters if it stays on the page.

So I encourage you: review the chapters again. Revisit your notes. Choose one area to focus on first and commit to taking action today—no matter how small it may seem.

For cancer patients: you are not alone

If you are currently living with cancer, please know this: you are not your diagnosis.

You are a whole human being with strength, dignity, and infinite value. You've taken the brave step of educating yourself, and that alone is empowering. Now, surround yourself with the tools, people, and mindset that will help you thrive—not just survive.

No matter the stage or prognosis, there is always room for healing—emotionally, spiritually, and often physically.

For caregivers and supporters: you are needed

If someone you love is battling cancer, this book has shown you how vital your role truly is.

You don't have to be a medical expert to be a healing presence. What matters most is your willingness to show up, listen without judgment, and offer steady, compassionate support. Sometimes the most powerful thing you can say is simply: "I'm here."

A vision for the future

When I began writing this book, I envisioned a world where:

- People knew how to prevent cancer before it starts

- Patients were empowered, not helpless

- Caregivers had clear tools and confidence

- Society no longer viewed cancer as a death sentence—but as a journey of transformation

That vision is no longer a dream—it can become reality. But it requires each of us to share, act, and uplift one another.

You now carry the power to make a difference, not only in your own life, but in your community, family, and the world.

Final words

What you know can spark awareness—but what you DO with what you know will create change.

So don't let these lessons stay inside a book. Bring them into your life. Share them with others. Start conversations. Support someone. Show up for yourself.

Let this moment mark the beginning of a new chapter—one where you are informed, intentional, and inspired to make the choices that support health, healing, and purpose.

And if you'd like to go deeper, I invite you to explore my programs at www.LifeBossHealth.com, where you'll find additional tools, hypnosis-based support, and guidance for cellular regeneration and emotional wellbeing.

Remember, you are not powerless. You are not alone. You are capable.

And above all, you are worthy of healing.

With all my support,

Dr. Lucy Coleman

Founder of LifeBoss Health®

Creator of the Hypnocell® Method

Appendix
Groups of carcinogens

(IARC classification)

The International Agency for Research on Cancer (IARC) continuously updates its list of agents classified based on the strength of evidence linking them to human cancer risk. As of June 27, 2025, they've evaluated 135 Group 1 agents (known carcinogens) and 95 Group 2A agents (probable) .

Group 1 – Carcinogenic to humans

These agents have sufficient evidence to cause cancer. Noteworthy additions in recent updates include automotive gasoline as Group 1, and gasoline additives like MTBE and ETBE classified as probable carcinogens (Group 2B) .

Key agents include:

- Tobacco smoking, secondhand smoke, and smokeless tobacco

- Processed meat, alcoholic beverages, acetaldehyde (in alcohol)

- Asbestos, silica dust, wood dust, diesel engine exhaust, outdoor air pollution

- Certain infections: HPV types (e.g. 16/18), hepatitis B and C, Epstein–Barr virus, HHV-8, H. pylori, liver flukes

- Ionizing radiation, solar UV, tanning devices, plutonium, radon

- Chemicals in industry: benzene, formaldehyde, benzidine dyes, vinyl chloride, 1,3-butadiene, cadmium, nickel compounds, polycyclic aromatic hydrocarbons

- Certain chemotherapy agents: cyclophosphamide, melphalan, etoposide

- Hormone drugs: tamoxifen, diethylstilbestrol (DES)

- Occupational exposures: mining, rubber manufacturing, painter, chimney sweep, coal tar, leather dust, etc.

Recent updates added: compounds like hydrochlorothiazide, voriconazole, tacrolimus recognized as carcinogenic to humans .

Group 2A – Probably carcinogenic to humans

These agents have limited human evidence and sufficient animal or mechanistic evidence. Examples:

- Red meat consumption, emissions from high-temperature frying

- Glyphosate (common herbicide), night-shift work

- Certain pathogens like HPV type 68, malaria (Plasmodium falciparum), and Merkel cell polyomavirus (MCV)

Why it matters?

- IARC classifies hazards, not actual risk—the probability of cancer depends on exposure level and individual susceptibility .

- New agents are continually reviewed. For example, gasoline was only recently upgraded to Group 1 in 2025; emerging substances like hair straightening products, GLP-1 analog drugs (e.g. Ozempic, Wegovy), and electronic nicotine devices are now on IARC's high-priority review list set for 2025–2029 .

Quick summary of updated dangerous categories:

- Group 1 (known carcinogens): Smoking, processed meats, asbestos, UV tanning, airborne pollutants (e.g. diesel exhaust), certain chemotherapy agents, viruses like HPV & hepatitis, benzene, formaldehyde, gasoline, s ilica.

- Group 2A (probable): Red meat, glyphosate, night-shift work, high-temp frying emissions, certain infections (HPV68, malaria), some occupational exposures.

About the author

Dr. Lucy Coleman is a renowned specialist in Human Reproduction and Embryology, with a lifelong commitment to integrative medicine, patient-centered care, and cellular health. Her career spans over two decades of international experience, during which she has traveled extensively, studying and designing comprehensive programs to enhance health, prevent disease, and promote lasting well-being.

Driven by a deep understanding of the challenges posed by chronic illnesses, Dr. Coleman has developed a unique healing approach that places patient empowerment at the center of recovery. This vision led her to create the LifeBoss Health®, a transformative health platform that combines cutting-edge science, mind-body techniques, and lifestyle medicine to support healing at the cellular level.

Early in her scientific journey, Dr. Coleman made a powerful observation: living cells are not only influenced by external factors, such as toxins or treatments, but also by the internal environment of thoughts, emotions, and subconscious beliefs. This insight became the foundation of her work in cellular regeneration—a discipline she has refined and practiced for years, yielding outstanding results for patients with cancer and other chronic conditions.

Her method blends advanced concepts in embryology, neuroplasticity, and epigenetics with hypnosis, visualization, and mental reprogramming, empowering patients to become active participants in their own recovery.

Dr. Coleman continues to share her groundbreaking work through books, courses, and public speaking. Her goal is to make this knowledge accessible to anyone facing the difficult path of illness, offering hope, clarity, and scientifically sound tools for transformation.

Explore more of her books on her Access her latest healing programs, cancer recovery courses, and guided meditation techniques for self-hypnosis and self-healing at www.LifeBossHealth.com.

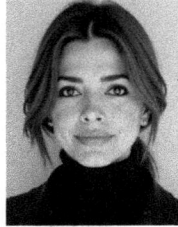

I would love to hear from you

Thank you for taking the time to read The Cellular Regeneration of Cancer. Writing this book has been a deeply personal journey—rooted in years of scientific research, clinical experience, and heartfelt conversations with patients navigating the challenges of cancer. My goal has always been to offer hope, insight, and empowerment to those seeking a deeper understanding of their healing potential.

If this book resonated with you in any way—if it brought you clarity, comfort, or a sense of renewed strength—I would be truly honored to hear your thoughts. Your feedback means the world to me, and it helps me continue refining this work to better serve others on similar paths.

Whether you're a patient, caregiver, or simply someone exploring the healing power of the mind and body, I invite you to share your story with me. Every case is unique, and I would be grateful to know how this book has touched your life or supported your process of transformation.

You can reach me directly through my website at or connect via my Amazon author page: .

Thank you again for reading. Remember, your body holds immense wisdom, and the journey of healing begins with trusting it.

With all my best, Dr. Lucy Coleman

www.ingramcontent.com/pod-product-compliance
Lightning Source LLC
Chambersburg PA
CBHW060853280326
41934CB00007B/1023